ANNA SHAPIRO

To Stephen & Carol
may the blessings of
God be with you
always. Joy Ashapi

GENTLE YOGA WITH
GREAT BENEFITS

For people who are in recovery, over

the age of 60, or have physical limitations.

2014

WARNING

Models for photos are Julia Babushkina and Victor DalPozzal.
Photographs by Cheryl DalPozzal
The editor: Susanne Kummel

ISBN 978-0-9860467-6-6
Library of Congress Control Number: 2014947905

Published by: Aspekt Publishing
Budget Printing Center
40 Weir St., Taunton, MA 02780
508-880-4729
www.budget-printing-center.com

ACKNOWLTDGEMENT

I first would like to acknowledge all the great masters before me, who were my inspiration and guiding light on my path to spirituality, especially Paramahansa Yogananda and Swami Kriyananda. Without their guiding Light the doors of self-realization would never have opened for me. I would like to offer a special thanks to the leaders and members of Ananda Spiritual Community in Nevada City, CA for the many years of support and guidance they have offered me in learning and deepening my roots in spiritual life. I am thankful that I was given a wonderful opportunity to help and heal people in this life.

My heart is full of love and gratitude to my husband Mark for giving me his complete support and great patience. I also owe a special debt of gratitude to my daughter Luba for inspiring me and bringing me spiritual and emotional support. I offer my appreciation to the rest of my family for believing in me while writing this book.

TABLE OF CONTENTS

INTRODUCTION

"The true purpose of yoga is to facilitate the development of Self-awareness–not as a self-enclosure, but as a doorway to an expanded awareness of the surrounding universe, of truth, of very life."

– Swami Kriyananda, from the book
Ananda Yoga for Higher Awareness

Yoga is a very ancient Indian system that is used for self-improvement on physical, emotional, and mental levels. The yoga system can be easily modified to cope with some physical limitations or health problem. It helps maintain better health, develop body flexibility, increase energy level, and cultivate emotional and mental calmness. In Sanskrit "Yoga" means *"Union,"* referring to harmony between body, mind and soul; union between a person's individual consciousness and spirit with the cosmic consciousness and spirit, or God.

Thousands of years ago, Yoga was developed as a system for self-development and self-healing. This book focuses on how people can help cope with such psychological issues as stress, lack of energy, depression and anxiety, as well as with physical problems and pain. It also discusses how yoga practice can help bring balance and increased energy for people of different ages as they recover from serious illnesses, or to those who have a disability. The book also focuses on self-healing for those who cannot attend regular or advanced yoga classes.

It is common that around 50–60 years of age, people usually begin to have less body flexibility, more muscle tension and joint stiffness, and they often become emotionally and mentally tired more easily. People of different ages who have disabilities can help and heal themselves by practicing easy yoga postures, breathing exercises and relaxation techniques. The aim of this book is to explain why it so important to learn and practice breathing exercises with deep relaxation and meditation— and to show that it is practically accessible for many people, from young to elderly, who have physical limitations and emotional problems.

We will spend much time talking about the psychological issues that affect how people feel about themselves. I emphasize that people should believe in themselves more than anybody else. I will show you how to develop and improve awareness of the personal problems that are affecting your life. It is up to each individual to improve self-control, and to appreciate his possibilities as well as his limitations. For example, how much can you stretch your body and how long can you hold the yoga posture? Yoga helps to develop self-control on all levels: physical, emotional and mental. It is also increases intuition.

In my personal life, yoga has helped me to survive physically and emotionally in the "dark" period in Soviet Russia and after my immigration to America. I was born right before WWII and from early childhood I experienced famine and malnutrition. I suffered from different serious illnesses, such as severe asthma, polyarthritis, and obesity, and at 20 years old I was on disability. When I was at school I was often ill and had to study at home. When I was 27, I joined a yoga group in which there were around 100 students. From the very first class I felt that this path was mine; I practiced yoga very seriously and with great interest. At the time, I had some physical limitations to doing the postures, so I did what I could. I paid more attention to the breathing and relaxation exercises. Thanks to yoga I changed my diet, stopped eating meat and gradually switched to vegetarianism. Once a week I fasted and drank only water. Slowly I lost a significant amount of weight. A year later many of my health problems were disappearing or at least were under control. I remember meeting my doctor on the street a couple of years after starting yoga; I had not seen him in a while. In the past, when he visited me at home, he used to say, "Unfortunately medicine cannot help you. I've done all that I can." Then he would leave. Seeing me on the street, happy, thinner and walking with ease, he stopped and said with surprise, "Is it really you? Are you still alive?" I did not know what to say in response but just thought to myself, "How wonderful that he is no longer my doctor." Thanks to yoga I became stronger physically and emotionally.

Some of the chapters are focused on a deeper understanding of such psychological issues as "Energy balance," "Stress," "Strength of mind," or "Pain relief." If you find that reading about these issues is not interesting to you, you can skip them and look further to the chapters that present practical yoga postures, relaxation, and breathing.

Love and self-respect are very important feelings. Follow the yoga principle: "I love myself for who I am." Realize that you do not need to be someone else. The paradox is that by accepting yourself the way you are, you then free yourself to change and become different. Only you are responsible for creating and maintaining your relationship with yourself. So be grateful and forgiving to yourself. Yoga will help you to be more conscious of life, physically more flexible and healthier, emotionally calmer and more balanced, and mentally you will feel more self-confident and strong.

Imbalance between body, mind and soul may lead to mental and physical fatigue, and this may be the cause of disease, pain or emotional problems. Yoga—including relaxation, breathing, light physical stretching, healing meditation, visualization, and healing prayer—will help you improve your health, grow mentally and emotionally stronger, and feel happiness and joy.

On the psychological level, the benefits of yoga are that it improves mood, increases self-confidence and attention, and that it can bring you to a spiritual level that helps reduce stress and anxiety. Yoga also helps answer very important philosophical questions about the meaning of life like *Who am I?* and *Why am I here?*

In our daily life we often function in a mundane way without being aware of many things about ourselves. Yoga can lead us through the development of a state of consciousness that includes an increased awareness, a sense of security, acceptance of our bodies, improved strength to accomplish our goals, and openheartedness. It helps us become spiritually aware in daily life.

If you have any back, neck, cardiovascular conditions, or other medical conditions you are aware of, it is extremely important that you get clearance and guidance from your doctor to do yoga.

Special attention is given to healing meditation and healing prayer for help resolving internal tension and conflicts. This book also may help the younger generation deal with stress, anxiety and any depression that holds them back.

Yoga Parable: The Shape of Things

There was once a famous sculptor. One day some people who wanted to see his work visited him. He took them to his studio and showed them a number of pieces of stone that had been partly chipped away. None of the stone blocks resembled anything tangible and were far from being beautiful. The visitors were a little disappointed, for they came expecting to see aesthetic pieces of sculpture. Then the sculptor said: "This is where I start work on my creations; now let us go to the next room." His visitors went to the next room and were confronted with objects that were beginning to look shapelier. They were more impressed. Then the sculptor led them to another room and showed them exquisite works of art. The visitors were delighted and exclaimed that they had never seen such delicate pieces of sculpture. But the sculptor explained that he had not finished work on them; they had yet to be polished before they reached the stage of perfection. The gradual transformation that the visitors saw in the sculptures is analogous to the

11

transformation that takes place in an individual when he practices yoga. At first his character is gross and rough. Something is lacking. Then in time his attitude towards life, himself and others changes. His sensitivity increases. He starts to radiate that which is already within him. Yoga unfolds the inner being of the individual, in the same way that the sculptor slowly exposes the shape of his works. The shape is already inherent within the stone – the sculptor only cuts away the extraneous material that hides it. In the same way, the inner potential of the individual always exists – yoga merely cuts away the dross to allow it to show itself. – Swami Satyananda Saraswati, "Yoga and Kriya"

ENERGY BALANCE

The most important goals of yoga are to increase and maintain energy level and to develop balance between body, mind and soul [2, 3, 5, 6, 12, 15, 17]. Any disease, as tells us, results from imbalances or blockages of vital energy in our bodies. By removing the blockage and stimulating the flow of energy, the body can naturally heal itself. Blocked energy becomes negative and can gradually become the cause of pain in different parts of the body. It's as if there is a river of energy trying to flow through the body but when the channels are blocked, the energy becomes immobile or stationary.

Ways to restore energy

Everyone can intuitively feel that in young and middle age when we get tired and lose energy, we can easily restore it. With age, after about 50 years, our bodies need more energy for everyday life because we spend more energy than we are able to accumulate it. There are many natural ways to restore energy, like being in nature, sleeping, listening to healing music, walking, swimming, etc. Yoga is one of the best ways to restore and save up life energy. Most, if not all, diseases manifest themselves first as a decrease of energy level and then appear as problems in the body.

When people under age 40 become tired, they can easily restore their energy level through physical exercise, sports, good sleep, and by feeling joy. The older we get, the more easily we lose energy because of the increased strain and stress at physical, emotional and mental levels—thus we have a greater difficulty restoring our energy level.

Qualities of energy: physical, emotional, and mental

Yoga teachings inform us that every person has different qualities of energy: physical, emotional, and mental. There is also a subtle energy, or the energy of the nerve cells. In yoga this is referred to as *prana*, a Sanskrit word that means "vital life force energy." Understanding this energy is the key to understanding the relationship between mind and body. Yoga teachings explain that poor health is a result of the fact that the subtle energy, or *prana*, is blocked, and thus the harmonious interaction between mind and body has become disturbed. For example, a tension headache is usually accompanied by blockages of subtle energy that can result in tension of the neck, shoulders and facial muscles. Blockages, containing negative energy, become a cause of emotional and physical tension. If the blockage lasts long enough it can lead to pain, discomfort, disease or exhaustion of the nervous system. Yoga teachings show us how to release negative energy by physical stretching, deep relaxation, breathing exercises, and meditation. When negative energy is released from a blockage it is transformed into positive, healing energy.

Subtle energy or "life force" sustains a person's life and health. There are three major sources of subtle energy or *prana*: solar prana, atmospheric prana, and prana of the earth.

Solar prana is sunlight. It revitalizes the body and stimulates good health. To accumulate solar prana you should to stay in the sun for five to ten minutes once or twice daily, or drink bottled water that was opened in sunlight. Prolonged exposure to too much solar prana may be harmful for the body because it is extremely strong.

From your own experience, you may remember how you felt when on a beach, standing on top of a mountain, or while walking through the woods and the sun suddenly filters down through the trees. You may have felt such an emotional elevation that you wanted to inhale more deeply and hold your breath. You may have felt a burst of energy and your soul filled with joy. These examples show that you gain subtle energy in your nerve cells, and at these moments, *prana*, or life force, freely flows in your body. Contact with nature is an effortless way to increase your energy level.

Prana contained in the air is called *atmospheric prana*. Breathing exercises, which will be described later, help to absorb more subtle energy from atmospheric air by using the full capacity of the lungs. Short shallow breathing uses only part of the lungs.

Subtle energy contained in the earth is called *earth prana*. It is absorbed through the soles of the feet. This happens automatically and unconsciously. So it is very useful to walk barefoot on the grass, sand, or water in good weather.

During bad weather, many people get sick not because of changes in temperature, but because of a reduction in solar and atmospheric prana. At such times many people feel mentally and physically sluggish or run the risk of getting viruses or encountering other health problems.

Yoga is a wonderful system that helps counteract this type of depletion in energy. It teaches us how to accumulate and save up prana that nourishes nerve cells all through the body. And this is vitally important for sustaining good health.

Accumulating positive energy through Yoga practice

Bringing more positive energy into your life and body is a skill, and like any new skill it can be developed through practice—in this case, yoga practice. In the next chapters I will present yoga exercises that include physical stretching, breathing, relaxation and meditation that are very helpful for increasing the level of positive energy in your body. Doing these exercises will help you reduce tension, release blocked negative energy and help you to develop a powerful and positive attitude in your life.

I'd like to tell about an experience that took place 40 years ago in Moscow when I attended an advanced yoga class. It is a good example of how negative energy can be unblocked and used for self-healing. One day at the end of the yoga class a woman came up to the teacher and began to speak with him rather anxiously. I, as usual, was sitting close to the teacher and so could hear the conversation. The woman said that doctors had found a cancerous tumor in her abdomen. She was told to come back in three months to check if the tumor was growing or not and after that they would determine whether surgery should be performed. The teacher looked very calm; he began to explain and instruct the woman as to how she could help herself. He said she needed to concentrate and meditate on white light and visualize white light filling her body and especially her abdomen. The teacher recommended that she do this for three hours a day. He warned her that in the beginning it would be difficult but she should not stop doing it, and that gradually a "vision" of white light would appear. He explained that any disease, and even more so cancer, develops "in darkness," i.e. where there is a lack of life energy, *prana*. He explained that while she concentrated she should also visualize the tumor shrinking in a powerful stream of white light; the darkness would decrease and eventually disappear. Three months later the woman came to the teacher again, this time with a smile, and told him that her doctor had done new tests, and he was very surprised when he saw that the tumor had shrunk considerably. The doctor questioned her as to what she had done but she told him nothing. The teacher strongly encouraged the woman to continue practicing this

18

meditation and visualization every day for a year. He promised that after that year of self-healing she would be completely healthy.

This story shows that self-healing is based on the belief that subtle energy, or life force, can control and improve our health. Positive and negative beliefs respectively influence our health and also every aspect of our life.

Protection from negative influences from within and around

It is very important to realize that problems and stress lie behind significant parts of human reality, and we must not avoid them, but try to be conscious of and understanding of what they are. There are several sources of both positive and negative influences. There exist "circles" around each human being, and problems arise in each circle constantly. **The first circle** is small and most important; this is a human being with his or her personality, intellect, emotions, health, mood, and personal successes and failures. **The second circle** contains one's family, friends, home, job, and everything else that is currently meaningful in one's life. The **third circle** includes the city and the country of one's residence, with all their negative and positive environments and events. The bigger, **fourth circle** includes the whole world and everything we know about it from books, radio and TV. Unfortunately in modern society, we are continually bombarded with mostly bad news about the world and the people in it. **The fifth circle** is the biggest, this is the universe. The full moon, new moon, sunspots, movement of the stars and meteorites, and other cosmic events affect one's life and health to some degree. Our minds and bodies are sensitive, and every person lives under many negative influences from all the circles around him or her. So it is important to realize that it is essential for each of us to learn how to defend ourselves from the negativities of the surrounding "circles" by creating inner strength, inner peace and power, and a feeling of freedom. Good health is a must. Yoga gives us a wonderful opportunity to learn a unique system for self-healing, and to sustain the balance and harmony between body, mind and soul.

STRESS

Stress is a common problem that affects our lives, health, and our relationships with people [1, 5, 11, 12, 21, 25, 29]. The word *stress* includes all types of suffering like muscle tension, irritability, anxiety, and depression. Stress has become a way of life for most people in the world. That would not necessarily be bad—it depends on how we cope with stress. People should try to find the causes of stress in their social world, in their family relationships, and in their own health.

The reasons for stress

The reasons for stress could be a serious disease, a lack of money, the loss of a job, our memories of difficult times, or offenses and insults in the past. If the period of stress is not long and the stress is not very strong, we can usually find our own way of adaptation. We adjust and we are able to overcome it or use it to escape from dangerous situations. Any major changes in our lives, positive or negative, can become a cause for stress.

How can we help ourselves get through and overcome emotional or physical suffering? Life is always full of difficulties and disappointments. From childhood, when we become aware of ourselves, we learn intuitively how to overcome difficulties by adjusting to the changes within and around us. Actually, stress is essential and needed in order to grow, to reach our full development, and it helps us to become stronger. Overcoming stress requires a strong will to overcome stress and a lot of courage and energy. Psychologists believe that life without stress is just not possible; some scientists believe that life without stress is also, well, stressful.

Sometimes we experience long, painful periods of stress and feel too overwhelmed to overcome it. But later, maybe even years later, this stress turns out to have been essential to our personal growth or to positive changes in our life. We need to learn to look at stress and life difficulties as challenges and opportunities rather than as obligations and obstacles. Yoga is a perfect and natural system; it teaches us how to control emotions and how to save up subtle energy, how to strengthen the will, and how to stay calm during trouble.

Here is a good example: A lecturer, explaining to his students what stress is and how to control it, raised a glass of water and asked, "How much do you think this glass of water weighs?" The answers ranged from 20 to 500 grams. The lecturer then explained, "The absolute weight does not matter; it all depends on how long I hold the glass of water. If I hold it for a minute, it is not a problem. If I hold it for one hour, I would begin to feel the heaviness in my hand. If I hold this glass for an entire day, I will need to call an ambulance. In each case it is the same weight, but the longer I hold it the heavier it becomes."

The same thing happens under long periods of stress. Sooner or later stress becomes a burden because it is too energetically and physically "heavy" and we are just not able to tolerate it. As with the glass of water, we have to put it on the table for a while and let the hand and arm rest before holding it up again. After a break, a little rest, we will be able to hold the weight again.

How to control emotions and how to save energy during stress

Studies show that feelings of stress and anxiety correlate with an increase of hormone secretion—generally adrenaline and cortisol—into the blood stream, which is designed to help prepare the blood vessels, heart and muscles to work intensively to overcome the cause of the stress. This natural reaction helps the body to cope with danger or get away from it—fight or flight. When the stressful situation ends or is removed, life and bodily functions return to a normal level.

When the stress lasts a long time or occurs frequently, the secretion of these hormones, also known as "stress hormones," is maintained at a consistently high level. When the physical and emotional stress does not end or cannot be removed, this chronically high level of stress hormones often leads to serious instability and imbalance in the body and eventually to disease.

The following fable gives a good example of one of the ways in which intense stress can cause a short, normal reaction of anger and resentment that then develops into a strong motivation for action.

A Chinese man rode in a wagon on a bone-chilling winter day. A woman also rode in the wagon with her child. She wrapped and warmed her child against the frigid weather, yet she herself was becoming so very cold that her lips began turning blue. The man suddenly stopped the cart and pushed the woman out onto the road. He left her and continued on with the child. The woman was furious that her child had been taken away! She started to scream and run after the wagon. As she ran the blood began to circulate through her frozen body. The color returned to her skin and her hands and feet warmed up. When she caught up with the cart, the man stopped and said, "Sit down! Now you will live!"

Short periods of anger can be a form of energy if directed to help encourage a person to be more active and strong. On the other hand, when anger becomes chronic, it can be dangerous to the body and develop into a source of disease. Sometimes anger enables us to find a way to overcome a problem or to get away from it. Almost everyone feels anxious occasionally. But when people have constant feelings of fearfulness, worry, tension and agitation that keep them "on alert," it will eventually produce chronic stress. Our reaction to stress depends on our personality. If we choose to, we can learn how to change our reactions to external stressors and to control our emotions.

Many Yogic techniques help enhance inner calmness, peacefulness and harmony, decrease anxiety and improve one's mood. Sometimes you can sense that your jaws are clenched, your abdominal muscles tensed, or you feel tense through the back, neck or shoulders. Tensed muscles become the reason for the development of blocks of negative energy that can end up causing psychological problems like anxiety, fear, depression, and self-doubt.

It is known that some diseases are caused by prolonged stress; chronic accumulation of stress and anxiety is harmful to the body and can be a reason for depression, clogged arteries, hypertension, heart disease, stroke, cancer, chronic fatigue, intestinal disorders, migraines, respiratory problems, and many other illnesses. Chronic fatigue and stress also affect concentration and memory, weaken the immune system and therefore can be the cause of many other serious diseases. Negative thoughts and expectations also create great stress in the body. Scientific studies have shown that this negativity in mind and emotions has a detrimental effect on the cells of the brain, creating constant tension in the body that doesn't allow for relaxing and healing.

It is very important to take a break for some period of time during a stressful situation and to find a little time for oneself. It is very good to do the gentle yoga stretching exercises described below, learn yoga relaxation, correct breathing, and meditation. This will help you to be emotionally strong and calm, and to improve your self-control and self-healing skills.

Psychologists say that our brain cannot distinguish between real threats and imaginary stressful situations, so every time a situation strikes us as dangerous, either in reality, in the mind, or in memory, the brain and central nervous system respond to it as to a real threat. For example, an overturned cup of tea to one person is nothing—she can remove it quickly and forget about it—while for someone else it can be very upsetting, and it will take her some time to calm down. In other words, unpleasant situations and our reaction to them can be disparate; it depends on our attitude toward stress and toward the people who have caused it and also in their reaction to us in this distressed state.

Three possible behavior reactions to stress

Doctor Andrew Weil [12] explains that there are two kinds of ways to cope with stress: *healthy* and *not-so healthy*. The healthy cope is when a person is able to adapt or adjust, consciously or unconsciously, to the stressful situation, and he continues to be in balance; so stress creates no serious consequences. *Healthy coping* is taking an active approach to solving a problem; or taking a different view of the problem, so it doesn't seem to be a problem anymore. It also involves positive actions like breathing, relaxation and meditation that we can use to reduce internal stress. Some people intuitively feel and know how to mobilize their inner strength and help themselves to achieve inner balance, and maintain inner peace. They are able to remain present and calm enough in the situation to observe it and observe themselves within it

– which despite our seemingly inherent desire to avoid discomfort, proves to be one of the most useful and calming ways to deal with difficult situations.

My next example gives you an idea of how to cope with stress in a healthy way. In the late 70s teaching yoga in Russia was officially prohibited and yoga teachers had to work illegitimately. A friend of mine, Maya, was a yoga teacher like me. People were easily drawn to her because she was an openhearted and open-minded person. She always taught her students to spiritual self-development. One day she was arrested, which resulted in a well-publicized court case in Moscow. She was convicted and sent to prison in the Far East for two years, to a place where people were sent for committing serious crimes. Her family, friends and colleagues were very sad because they were not allowed to correspond with her. We didn't have any information from or about her.

I had also been teaching yoga illegally, so the following two years were very intense and fearful for me. One day the doorbell rang. When I opened the door I saw Maya. We hugged each other heartily; I could not believe my eyes—she looked very good and her eyes shone with happiness. She told me her story. In prison she was put in a cell with six other women who had committed real crimes in their past. From the first day Maya began to teach them yoga: breathing exercises, relaxation, physical stretching and postures; she taught them how to be emotionally strong and calm, and she also taught them how to increase their vitality and strengthen their will in order to overcome their current difficulties. Two years later Maya was released but these women had longer sentences than she had. They said goodbye to her in tears, expressed to her that they had been changed by her teachings and they now knew how to enjoy their lives even while living in prison.

What helped Maya to protect herself actively during such a long period of stress? And what helped her develop self-control in such a difficult situation? As she told me, practicing yoga helped her change her life and move from passivity to activity, using methods of conscious and active self-control and self-healing. The spiritual part of yoga helped her very much: relaxation, meditation, repetition of positive affirmations and deep yogic breathing helped her keep her mind and emotions calm and positively strong. Spiritual yoga techniques increase natural adaptability on both the mental and physical levels.

Unhealthy coping includes repressing or denying the stress-inducing problem, or just wishing it would go away. Instead of dealing with the problem, some people are constantly preoccupied with getting away from it. Another example of unhealthy coping with emotions is blaming others for one's problems.

Most stress comes from the desire to see things not as they are in reality. Mental and emotional anxiety increases stress. Sooner or later the stressful situations will be gone, but we often continue to experience the mental and emotional tension, or we continue to feel hurt by a past offense or event. So it is very important to find a little time for ourselves during the day, around 30 minutes, ideally, to do simple stretching, practice one or two breathing exercises, deep relaxation, and meditation; in addition to these it is very good to find a hobby that will fulfill you and make your life more interesting.

Why do people cry? A wise man said: When people are unhappy with each other and quarrel, their hearts are isolated. In order to cover the distance and hear each other, they have to shout. The angrier they get, the louder they shout. So, when arguing, do not let your hearts be disconnected from each other, do not speak words that will increase the distance between you and someone else. Because someday the conflict may become so great and serious that you will not be able to find a way back. People usually suffer a lot because of difficult relationships with others.

Here is an excerpt from a talk by *Nayaswami Anandi:*

As a disciple of Paramahansa Yogananda for more than 40 years, I have witnessed many miracles in my own life and in the lives of friends. I learned of a prayer by Paramahansa Yogananda that seems specially empowered to bring miracles of healing to anyone having conflicts with others. The prayer is quite simple: If you are having challenges with another person, visualize that person in light and for one minute pray: "Lord, fill him or her with peace and harmony, peace and harmony." Then visualize yourself in light and pray for 15 seconds: "Lord, fill me with peace and harmony, peace and harmony." The prayer also came with these additional words: "Do this 5 times a day — 3 or 4 times might work, but 5 times practically never fails.

Yoga techniques to control and release stress

Paramhansa Yogananda [3] said that life is nothing if not a continuous overcoming of problems. Every problem that waits for a solution at your hands is a religious duty imposed upon you by life itself.

Regular exercise and relaxation increase self-confidence and lower the symptoms related to stress, such as mild depression and anxiety [16, 17]. They improve your sleep, which is often disrupted by stress. Yoga can ease your stress levels and give you a sense of wellbeing, safety and happiness.

I'd like to present a fable called "Angry Words" that is a good illustration of what was said above.

Once, Buddha was passing through a village. One angry young man went up to him and began to be rude and insulting to him. "You have no right to teach others," - he cried. "You rascal! And you are as much a fool as everyone else." Buddha was not upset. Instead he asked the young man: "Tell me, if you buy a gift for someone, and the person will not accept it, to whom does the gift belong?"

The young man was surprised by such a strange question and answered: "It belongs to me because I bought it."

Buddha smiled and said: "Yes. In the same way, that's what happens when you are angry. If you are mad at me, but I do not get insulted and offended, then the anger falls back on you. Therefore, only you yourself become unhappy, not me. All that you have said has hurt only yourself. If you want to stop harming yourself, you must get rid of your anger and instead become loving.

This is also a good Japanese saying:

No door leads to happiness or unhappiness. Both enter in when you ask them to.

PAIN RELIEF

What is pain and how does it occur?

Yoga as presented in this book helps the whole body, not just a part of it. When a person suffers from chronic pain, his body changes, and to treat only the part that is in pain is not enough.

Everyone feels pain in different parts of the body sometimes. Pain is always uncomfortable, and if the pain occurs often or it is quite strong, you feel not only muscle tightness but also emotional and mental tension. Any kind of pain is a sign that our body is calling out to us: "Please pay attention to me." It is very important to be aware of and bring attention to yourself—to stop sometimes in the stream of the life and focus your mind on your body, emotions, and on your life as a whole.

Practicing yoga helps you to look within and find the ability for self-healing and the prevention or reduction of pain. To take responsibility for self-healing requires strength of will, self-control and self-discipline. When pain is strong you become more vulnerable and sometimes even angry. It is very important to believe in natural methods that can be used in combination with medical approaches for relieving pain. Yoga is one of the best systems of self-

34

healing but its effectiveness depends on your level of knowledge, patience and persistence in practicing it.

Medications are based on scientific studies, and although these studies are very important, they seldom result in complete healing. There are areas of human nature that science can never explain and treat: morality, love, will power, and soul. Each of us is a harmony—a unity of body, mind and soul—so it is very important to be aware of nature or, at least, of your personality as a whole. The mind and body interrelate all the time and much of this subtle connection happens at a subconscious level.

It is very important and necessary to use the achievements of medicine for relieving pain. One may hope and, indeed, there is little doubt that the study of the relationship of the three elements–body, mind, and soul—will be the future of medicine. People need help in learning how to achieve balance in the whole body, and yoga helps to attain such a balance, improve self-control and learn self-healing methods.

Types of pain

There are two types of pain, acute and chronic. An example of acute pain can be any type of trauma such as a cut, burn, or any time when pain is sharp and intense.

Chronic pain may occur frequently or rarely, it can be continual or dull; it depends on the sensitivity of the affected part of the body. Examples of chronic pain can be headaches, lower back pain, or arthritis pain.

Scientists have found that our brain produces natural anesthetic agents called endorphins that decrease pain [15, 22]. Endorphins block the sensation of pain and support well-being. The quantity of endorphins is different in each body and it is used according to the individual. Practicing yoga can increase the level of endorphins in the brain. Indeed regular physical activities like swimming, running, exercise, and especially yoga stretching postures increase the production of endorphins in the brain. More endorphins are also produced if a person has a positive mental attitude, experiences a feeling of fulfillment and pleasure, can engage in deep relaxation or meditation, and gets good, deep sleep.

This book does not deal with acute pain and especially pain in the internal organs such as the heart, liver, or kidneys, because these problems always require medical intervention and a doctor's treatment.

Pain can sometimes indicate the beginning of some illness which could be the result of a weakening of the vital forces in the body due to prolonged mental, emotional or physical stress, long chronic disease, or fatigue. This happens when a person has not paid enough attention to resting during a period of emotional strain and overwork.

Self-healing, preventing and decreasing pain

When you are in pain, you usually seek help by visiting a doctor to find out the reason for you pain. You can often wind up taking painkillers. You also can use methods such as physical therapy, acupuncture, herbs, massage, and sometimes get the help of a chiropractor or homeopath. All these healing approaches are very important and beneficial—they bring relief and ease the pain for a while, and maybe completely. But when you finish some of these treatments, it is the best time to continue to help yourself by practicing yoga, doing stretching exercises, deep relaxation, breathing exercises, and meditation with healing prayer, all of which are described below.

What is pain? How does it come up? It is commonly understood that our mind and body are in constant contact and interaction. The brain has unconscious defense mechanisms that have been widely studied by scientists and doctors at the Mayo Clinic in Minnesota in recent years [13]. They found the psychological causes of chronic pain and that pain usually occurs as a result of the three following processes:

The first process involves a person living under pressure or constant, unpleasant influences. Here, psychological stress is caused by internal factors, such as health problems, a long sense of grievance, feelings of guilt, or experiencing constant negative emotions like fear, anxiety, hate, and painful memories. External factors include for example, having to deal with difficult and annoying people in the family, at work, with neighbors or in other situations.

The second process has to do with the development of anger, emotional irritation, a feeling of stress or frustration that is a result of unpleasant pressure from outside and inside. Unfortunately, people are often not aware of these feelings and so they cannot get rid of them. As a result, all these negative emotions are unconsciously suppressed and forced into the subconscious. In psychology, suppression and repression of negative emotions are the protective functions of the brain to free up the mind. Thus, these functions are vital mechanisms of the brain because without them we could easily go mad. These suppressed and repressed negative emotions accumulate and form blocks of negative energy (as described above in "Energy Balance").

In *the third process,* blocks of negative energy can become a cause of health problems because the subconscious mind releases negative energy and sends it into different parts of the body, for example to the autonomic nervous system, which controls digestion, respiration, circulation and other involuntary body functions. This negative energy usually gathers in the so-called weak points of our body and can decrease blood flow to certain muscles, tendons and nerves, and to the brain, spine, and joints. These "weak" parts of the body become weaker and more sensitive, the body begins to suffer from reduced blood flow and oxygen to tissues, and all of these become a cause of pain. Yogananda said in one of his lectures: "We can be in pain, but suffering is our choice."

To prevent suffering you can learn and use these yoga self-healing exercises in everyday life. Gentle yoga as presented in this book is accessible to many people who are in pain or have disabilities because of physical and emotional problems.

The three most common types of pain— headache, low back pain, and arthritis pain are considered below.

Yoga for relief of headaches

Headache [3, 15, 22, 23, and 24] may occur infrequently and it can be associated with fatigue after a busy day at work, or the flu, or a bad pillow when the muscles of your neck are strained during sleep. Sometimes people experience repeated headaches. Chronic headaches gradually weaken one's physical and emotional health. Studies show that people who suffer from migraines are three times more likely to suffer from depression. Medications help temporarily but they often have side effects. Some people would rather avoid taking medications to prevent dependence on them.

Approximately 90 percent of all chronic headaches are tension headaches or migraines, or a combination. Psychological stress and negative emotions, plus fatigue and exhaustion, can lead to many physical problems.

The neck and the upper back are the most important parts of the body that need to be kept relaxed and flexible to prevent headaches. Many people, under stress, unconsciously tense their neck, facial and forehead muscles, and also the muscles of their shoulders and chest. These lead to tension in the brain vessels that can lead to spasms and pain.

Yoga presents natural methods for relief of headache pain that can be a very good addition to medical treatment if that is needed. The natural, preventive self-healing system, described below under, "Warm-Up Exercises," is a program of yoga stretching postures that can be done in lying position, sitting on a chair or in a standing position; deep muscle relaxation, breathing exercises, positive self-suggestions or affirmations, and also healing meditation and healing praying. Yoga tells us that you can prevent and lessen headaches with breathing exercises alone if they are done correctly. Yoga exercise is designed to improve your flexibility; it can also provide pain relief and gives a person a feeling of happiness.

Yoga postures for relieving back pain

According to statistics lower back pain [3, 15, 22, 23, and 24] is the second most frequent pain after headaches. It can result from different causes. Although the human spinal column is a structure of perfect engineering design, it is extremely vulnerable to the effects of stress and various physical overwork. The spinal column has important functions, it:

Supports the head and strengthens the skeleton;
Keeps the body in a vertical position;

Protects the spinal cord where nerves pass;

Provides the connection of the brain with other parts of the body;

Serves as a place of connection for muscles and ribs;

Enables the body to perform a variety of movements.

The most common causes of back pain are bad posture, weak abdominal muscles, incorrect weight lifting, or attempts at bodybuilding that involve workouts that are too intense or difficult. Lack of even a little physical activity also can lead to a reduction in flexibility, a decrease in the strength and endurance of the back muscles, and as a result, pain.

The spine is held in an upright position only by the lumbar muscles. They become weaker without regular physical activity, and as a result they are unable to keep the spine in an upright position. The practice of yoga postures is important mostly because it increases strength, flexibility and the function of the back muscles, and thus decreases the causes of pain. Without such regular practice, even a little, back muscles become too weak, and the very simplest movements can cause pain.

The abdominal muscles are like a corset, holding the abdominal organs close to the spine. A weakening of the abdominal muscles can be the result of a lack of physical activity and a passive lifestyle. Obesity can increase the weight on the lumbar spine. All these can bring excessive deflection of the lumbar, which ultimately leads to chronic back pain. In addition to yoga postures, it is very important to practice deep relaxation that stimulates production of the natural endorphins in the brain that reduce pain.

Physical therapy can really help if you have serious problems with your back. After a course of physiotherapy you should continue doing gentle yoga stretching and postures, breathing exercises, deep relaxation, and meditation; these all are very useful and helpful. If it is difficult for you to do yoga postures, you can practice just the breathing, relaxation and meditation at any time.

To maintain a healthy spinal column it is important to stretch your body in different directions, bending your spine forward and backward, twisting your body to the side and tilting to the left and right. Explanations of how to do it and photos of the postures are presented below.

Arthritis and emotional stress

The term "arthritis" [13, 15, and 24] literally means joint inflammation. Some forms of arthritis cause only minor problems and do not interfere with normal life. Others may affect the whole life of a human being. But almost all kinds of arthritis are chronic. Typical symptoms of arthritis are pain, morning stiffness, joint swelling with redness and hot skin, limited mobility in one or more joints or in the spine, or deformity of the joints over time. If you have such symptoms a rheumatologist must treat you.

Arthritis may be the oldest of the diseases known to mankind. It was discovered in a study that Egyptian mummies had arthritis; prehistoric man and dinosaurs also suffered from arthritis. Almost 40 million Americans suffer from arthritis. Many animals also have this disease.

Joint arthritis can be caused by traumatic injuries as well as by a variety of diseases caused by bacteria or viruses. Arthritis may be due to problems of the nervous system as well, such as severe emotional stress, depression, or metabolic disorders.

Arthritis in the knees is a common problem. Usually it occurs because of constant over-exertion, for example, over-tension or a cold. The most efficient therapy for arthritis is physiotherapy, which can include heat treatment,

44

magnetic therapy, massage, and acupuncture. Various Chinese physical exercises (qigong, tai chi, etc.) are also very good for the joints and muscles. Many doctors think that yoga is the most helpful for arthritis because it can be practiced every day. Do not forget that all exercises should be performed with caution and only after consultation with your doctor.

Chronic arthritis is often accompanied by emotional stress that can reduce resistance to the disease. Perhaps the worst effect of stress is increased muscle tension in different parts of the body that may intensify pain; this, in turn, becomes the root of feelings of helplessness and anxiety that can lead to depression. Thus a cycle is formed: stress, depression, increased pain and around again. But when you learn to be aware that you are under stress, it becomes possible to interrupt this cycle. It is important to recognize the following symptoms of stress: fatigue (which may be chronic), low mood, muscle tension, pain, worry, and anxiety.

Depression should be treated. If it is difficult for you to cope with depression, please see a doctor and take prescribed antidepressant medications for a while. When your mood improves you will be able to maintain your health and mood more easily by practicing yoga. Mild depression is often cured by increased physical activity because physical exercise increases production of serotonin in the brain. Serotonin is the natural drug that cures depression.

As for arthritis, even doing just a little stretching and yoga exercises promote joint flexibility and helps prevent pain. American doctors say that movement for arthritis can cause pain but inactivity may kill. Incorrect movement hurts, reasonable movement heals. Many doctors think that practicing yoga is the key to healthy joints. People with arthritis should practice it within their own limits as the disease allows; however, do not let the disease make you withdraw from all movement.

Recent research convinces us of the value of a psychological approach for the relief of pain related to arthritis. Some doctors recommend "hurrying slowly," in other words, learning to move at your own pace, and not trying to do too many physical activities when you feel good because it can lead to tiredness, pain or fatigue later on. Therefore, it is better to do a little yoga exercise every day regardless of whether you feel bad or good.

It is well known that swimming helps tremendously—releasing muscle tension and decreasing arthritis pain. The body in water becomes more relaxed and flexible, and this stimulates the release of endorphins, the natural painkilling substances in the brain. All water exercises must be done under the supervision of specialists. Doing some yoga stretching in a swimming pool increases the flexibility of the joints and vertebra. Breathing exercises and deep relaxation as described below also help to relieve muscle tension.

Yoga stretching for relieving arthritis pain and for joint flexibility

Arthritis, particularly the rheumatoid variety, makes you more vulnerable to fatigue. So when you feel tired it is crucial to rest, you should not push yourself. It is very important to listen to your body, understand it and trust the sensations coming from within. Be aware of both your own possibilities and limitations. Get in a nap during the day—sleep is the best rest. Practicing gentle yoga for self-healing helps keep arthritis under control and helps you believe in what you are doing.

Here are some simple stretching exercises to relieve finger stiffness and improve foot and ankle flexibility if you practice them daily:

1. Slowly curl the index finger by bending the middle joint until the tip of your index finger touches the uppermost part of you palm (Photo 1).

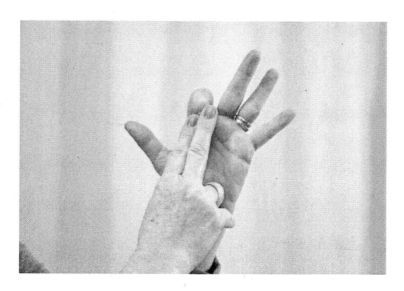

Photo 1

You can help move the finger with your other hand, if need be. Hold this position several seconds. Curl and uncurl other fingers in turn. Then move all four fingers simultaneously, curl and uncurl them.

2. Thumb Stretching. Open your hand, keep fingers straight and wide apart, extend your thumb away from your other fingers as far as you can. Then reach your thumb across your palm and try to touch your little finger (Photo 2). Hold this pose for a few seconds.

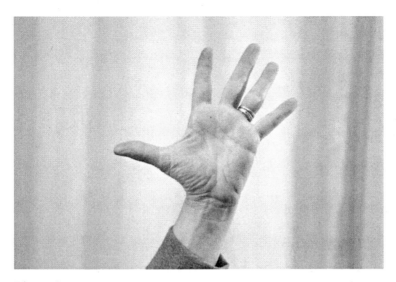

Photo 2.

3. Make a circular motion with your wrists in one direction and then the other.

4. To strengthen elbows and shoulders, raise your arms, straighten them on the sides and twist them, holding the position for several seconds, and then return to the initial pose (Photo 3). Repeat 2-3 times.

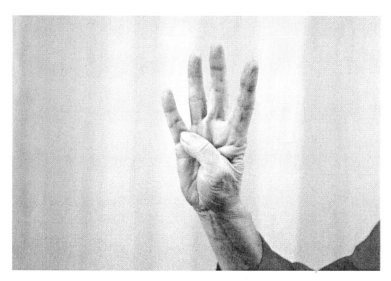

Photo 3.

Stretching feet and ankles: You can do these exercises lying on your back or sitting on a chair.

    5. Rotate your ankles so that your toes point in, toward each other (Photo 4a). Hold this position briefly.

    6. Rotate your ankles in the opposite direction, pointing your feet outward (Photo 4b). Hold briefly.

    7. Sit on a chair. Use your ankles to swivel your feet, first on tiptoe (Photo 5a), then on your heels (Photo 5b). Try to hold each position for 3-5 seconds.

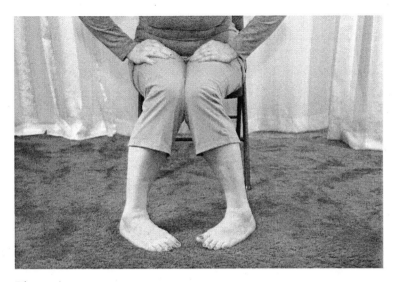

Photo 4a.

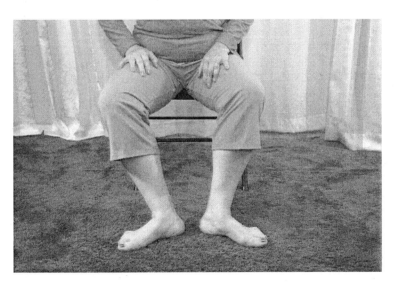

Photo 4b.

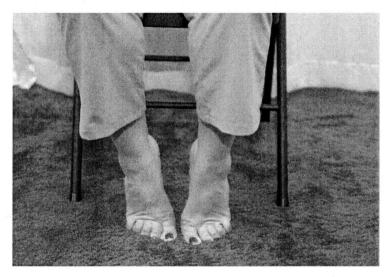

Photo 5a.

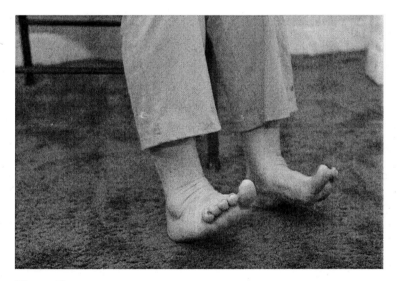

Photo 5b.

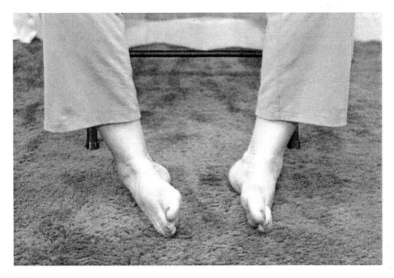

Photo 5c.

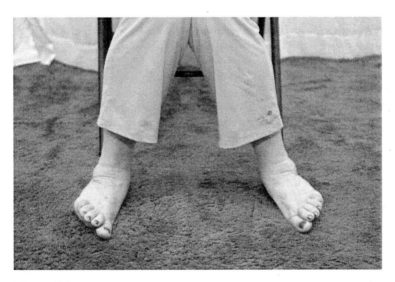

Photo 5d.

8. Side Stretches: Lift your arches a little, but don't lift your feet off the floor, so that the soles of the feet face each other (Photo 5c). Then put your feet back on the floor and roll onto your arches with your soles facing out (Photo 5d). Your ankles should be doing all the work.

People with arthritis feel better when they rest and stay calm. But long rest can increase stiffness and can be the cause of muscle weakness. During acute illness and severe pain bed rest is recommended. Only you can decide how long you need to rest and how much and how long you should exercise. Even with a doctor's help, you should learn to listen to and understand your own body.

Each person suffering from arthritis has his own individual degree of mobility, so choose the yoga postures, described below, according to your individual experience, capability and limitations. You should look over all the exercises in "Warm-Ups" and in "Yoga Postures," and then choose those that are best suited to your health condition.

If you have serious health problems you should see your doctor and discus with him what exercises and postures you could do from yoga.

If you are in the process of recovery, begin practicing yoga postures slowly in a lying position and do them for 1-3 weeks. Pay attention to your body and to your reactions, do not force the movement, and do not push

54

yourself. Then, when you feel better and have more energy, you can begin to do postures while sitting on a chair over a period of 1-3 weeks. And after that try to practice yoga poses in standing position near a wall.

If you find out that you are not yet ready for yoga postures, practice light exercises for your hands and feet, or some exercises from the "Warm-Up" section that follows. Every day, practice deep relaxation, breathing exercises, and, if you feel ready, meditate with healing prayer. These practices are very accessible for nearly everyone in any condition of health.

In the previous section, we have discussed three types of pain, plus how to prevent and decrease headaches, back pain and arthritis pain. For more than 30 years, scientists have been conducting research that shows how deep relaxation and meditation can stabilize blood pressure, reduce heart rate, and decrease emotional stress.

Yoga for eyes:

Strengthening and Improvement

Our eyes are windows into the world and our perception of the world, in many respects, depends on the eye health. In fact, vision occupies about forty percent of the brain's capacity. That is why we close our eyes in order to relax and fall asleep. Vision problems arise with age from a gradual loss of flexibility and resilience in the eye muscles. Yogic health covers all aspects of human life, including the strengthening and improvement of vision. Yoga offers specific and easy exercises for the eyes that should be practiced preferably daily for 5-10 minutes. These exercises are very beneficial for improving vision, but especially they are useful for those who have nearsightedness, farsightedness and astigmatism. According to Swami Sitaramananda, director of the Sivananda Yoga Vedanta Center of San Francisco, "The fastest way to bring the mind into concentration is through the eyes." You should do the exercises sitting on a chair in a comfortable position with a straight back.

Exercise 1

Sit quietly with eyes closed and take a few deep breaths to help you relax completely. Concentrate your gaze on one object for 3-4 minutes: you may look at an apple on the table, or at a dot on the wall in front of your eyes at a distance of 1 - 1.5 meters, or gaze on a flame of a burning candle placed at eye level. Look attentively at the middle of the flame or an object. Try not to blink too much. Keep muscles of the eyes and face relaxed. Then close your eyes and try to maintain a vivid mental image of the object you were concentrating on, for as long as possible. Repeat in this manner a few times according to your comfort level. Each time you practice, try to extend the time you maintain the mental after-image. Breathe calmly and rhythmically. This is a very effective exercise and provided beneficial effects not only for your vision, but also significantly improves concentration, attention, increases efficiency and mental fortitude; thoughts become calmer and clearer.

Exercise 2

Close your eyes and with fingertips gently tap on your eyelids, then rub the palms of your hands vigorously, until they become warm. Then place cupping your palms gently over your eyelids. Relax your eyes and eyelids, while becoming aware of warm feel of energy emanating from the palms. Maintain calm and rhythmic breath. Hold this position for a few seconds or as long as you prefer. This exercise is also beneficial when your eyes are tired.

Exercise 3

Sitting on a chair keep your back straight. Relax and breathe quietly. Look as far to the left as possible without moving your head and hold for a second. Then repeat looking to the right, while moving your eyes in a horizontal line, and hold for a second. Follow this exercise with horizontal eye movements ending with "palming" (cupping your hands over your eyes), 2-nd exercise. Then look up and down holding each position for a second. Repeat this exercises 10 times. Then close your eyes and relax. Don't move your head; keep your head, neck and chest on the one line.

Exercise 4

Now look along the diagonal: to the upper left corner, and then to the lower right corner. Then look to opposite diagonal: to the upper right corner and then to the lower left corner. Repeat movements of your eyes along diagonals several times.

Exercise 5

Now begin shifting your focus between the tip of the nose and the faraway point. Pause at each point for one-two seconds. Repeat the exercise 10 times, and then relax your eyes with palming and deep breathing. Finish by closing your eyes and relaxing.

Exercise 6

Sit with your back straight. Visualize a big circle in front of you. Follow an edge of the imaginary circle with your eyes only, first a few times in one direction, and then in the opposite direction. Close and relax your eyes when you are done. After finishing all exercises, repeat the 2nd one: close your eyes and gently tap with your fingertips on the eyelids, then rub your hands together and put them over your eyelids. Breathe and relax.

Practicing these exercises regularly for a few months can go a long way in facilitating the normal functioning of your eyes. Yoga teaching offers these simple exercises for strengthening of vision. According to Robert Abel, author of The Eye Care Revolution, these brief exercises "compensate for overdevelopment of the muscles we use to look at near objects."

BREATHING

What does breath mean for us? With each inhalation the lungs and body take in oxygen, and with each exhalation the lungs emit carbon dioxide. Yoga also teaches us that breathing is a source of subtle energy, *prana*, or the vital life force of the body [3. 6]. Breath is the bridge, a connection between mind, emotions and bodies, and their functions. When we pay attention to our breath and watch for it, our awareness is drawn into the body and the mind shifts to focusing on the breath. When the mind and body achieve integration and balance, we become "embodied" and experience a sense of our intrinsic wholeness and unity. The breath is like a barometer that reflects our state of mind, our well being and our experience in every moment of our lives. In turn, our thoughts and emotions also affect our breath. When we have negative thoughts and experience panic, anxiety or become overly excited, our breath becomes rapid and shallow.

Yoga offers different kinds of breathing exercises, which have a positive effect on the body. Some of them bring heat and energy into the body; and when we focus our mind through breathing we may also have a cooling effect on the body. Specific breathing exercises clean the nostrils, calm you, create balance, and release tension in the body and mind.

Focusing on breathing while doing the yoga postures allows us to be aware of our body conditions at each moment and stay tuned and listen to any positive changes. The body gives us feedback as to how deeply to go into the posture, what subtle shifts we need to make, and when to come out of the pose. Breathing exercises should be done in sitting position with a straight back, and the head, the neck and the chest should be kept in alignment with one another. Clothing should be loose. In the beginning, if you have difficulties doing the breathing exercises while sitting on a chair, you may do them lying on your back. Breathing exercises should be done one hour before a meal, 3-4 hours after a large meal, or 1-2 hours after a light meal.

Concentrate on your breathing and feel the flow of air through your nostrils. Breathe silently while relaxing your facial muscles and the muscles of your nose and throat. While doing the breathing exercises concentrate also on the movements of your diaphragm, rib cage and upper chest. Breathe consciously. An Indian saying that is very apt explains: The way we breathe is the way we live. There are many breathing exercises in yoga but I have chosen three of them because they are the most important and can easily be learned by everyone.

Calming Breathing

Calming breathing is naturally diaphragmatic, and rhythmic. This kind of breathing is natural for newborns and for everyone in sleep. All animals breathe from their diaphragm as well. In the beginning, it is easiest to learn while you lie on your back with bent knees and your hands placed on your abdomen. After some practice, you will be able to breathe in this calm way while you are sitting or standing as well.

Now lie on your back, close your eyes and just watch how the air in your breath comes in and goes out. Consciously let go of tension, and then feel that your breathing is getting calmer. Focus your mind on the navel and watch how it moves up and down as you breathe in and out. Yoga teaches us that the navel is the center of our physical body, and when we concentrate the mind on it, breathing naturally becomes quiet. Breathe in and out only through the nose. With each inhalation slightly push your abdominal muscles out, and as you exhale draw abdominal muscles in. Breathe without effort, naturally, and when exhaling, feel yourself letting go of all the general tension in your body. Focus your attention solely on the movement of your abdominal muscles and do not raise your chest and shoulders. Practice this breathing for 3-5 minutes and gradually, day by day, it will become your habitual way of breathing. Learn to breathe calmly and rhythmically from your diaphragm everywhere during the day and you will feel that it helps you to maintain calmness, energy balance, and peace of mind. Calming breathing is very good to practice especially before going to sleep. It helps you sleep more deeply, and in the morning you wake up with more energy and feeling more refreshed.

It is very useful to practice diaphragmatic breathing for stretching the lower lobes of the lungs. Keep practicing calm, rhythmical breathing anytime and anywhere.

Full Deep Yogic Breathing

Deep, long breathing is important and useful, not only for your lungs on a physical level, but also as a means of increasing and balancing *prana*. The action of breathing deeply, inhaling oxygen and exhaling carbon dioxide, becomes a source of "life force" or "vital energy"—in other words, it is a source of subtle energy, *prana,* which as I said above is "food" for the nerve cells of the brain. There are three phases of full, deep yogic breathing: lower, middle, and upper breathing. Slow, deep inhalation and exhalation should be smooth, without pauses between the phases because these steps are conditional. The *first* phase is breathing from your diaphragm; the **second** phase involves movement of the ribcage muscles—their expansion in the front, sides and back. Yoga teachings inform us that emotionally uptight and mentally tense **people have** too much tension in the muscles between their lateral ribs. People who are able to breathe easily, expanding their rib muscles, have more courage and have a wider view of the world. In the *third* phase of deep breathing, the upper part of the chest rises. In the beginning, take some time to learn to breathe in each phase separately and feel the movement of the muscles of your diaphragm, then the ribcage, and then the upper chest.

The lower breath is diaphragmatic. That is the one described above as "Calming Breathing." The second, middle phase is the expansion of the ribcage. Put your hands on the side of your ribs and feel your ribcage expand as you inhale. As you exhale, put slight pressure on your ribs with your hands and feel the air coming out. While doing this exercise, try to not move your diaphragm or your upper chest—focus your movement and attention exclusively on the middle area of your torso. For the third phase of deep full breathing, the upper level, feel the upper area of the lungs and chest expand and move up as you inhale, and then sink again as you exhale.

Eventually, all three parts of full breathing merge smoothly into one another. In the beginning it is better to practice full breathing while lying on your back because it is easier to feel how the air is filling your lungs. Then with practice you will be able to do this exercise sitting on a chair.

Sit on a chair, breathe normally, relaxing your shoulders, chest and abdominal muscles. Keep your back upright and your spine straight. Now expel all the air out of your lungs. Then expand the diaphragm as you breathe in, now feel the expansion of your rib muscles, and then continue to inhale, raising your upper chest. Pay most attention to the middle phase because the more your rib cage expands the more air you are able to inhale. Breathe in as deeply as you can. It takes some time and practice to bring awareness to all three phases as you breathe in. Exhale slowly and freely in the reverse direction. It is also important to feel that your inhalation and exhalation are equal in length.

It will be easier if you mentally count to six as you inhale and to six again as you exhale. If you find it difficult and you start to feel tension trying to breathe in and out to six, change the rhythm and count to four instead. Gradually your breathing will become slower and deeper. Each person has an individual rhythm. To find out what rhythm is best for you, check your pulse, remember its rhythm, and then use it in your mental count as you inhale and exhale. In the beginning do at least seven cycles (one cycle consists of both inhaling and exhaling). If it is difficult to do seven cycles in a row you may take a rest between cycles and, while you are resting, breathe naturally in a relaxed way.

Full yogic breathing has a great effect on all levels of the body: physical, emotional, mental, and spiritual. Deep, long breathing fills your body with energy, improves the immune system, strengthens the lungs and heart, calms the nervous system, relieves mental and emotional stress, reduces anxiety, and improves mood. Practicing such breathing helps develop the ability to achieve emotional and mental self-control and to be healthier on all levels.

Alternate Nostril Breathing

For this breathing exercise your fingers must be in the correct position. The index and middle finger of the right hand are folded over and pressed against the middle of the palm. Extend the thumb, the ring finger and little finger (Photo A). The thumb is used to close the right nostril and

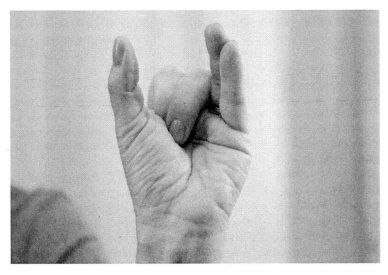

Photo A.

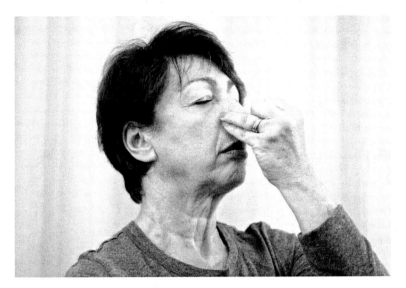

Photo B

the ring and little fingers together close the left nostril. Close your eyes and relax your facial muscles.

Now close the right nostril with your thumb, inhale through the left nostril slowly and deeply. Now close the left nostril with the ring and little fingers and open the right nostril, breathing out through it slowly and smoothly. Then inhale through the right nostril. Now close the right nostril and open the left nostril and exhale slowly. This is one round of alternate breathing. If you feel comfortable, practice three to five rounds in a row. But if you are tired and feel any discomfort in breathing, do only one round, rest, then do one more round. Focus your attention on the air coming through your nostrils. Slowly, with practice, you will be able to do more rounds and you will benefit a lot.

There are some easy variations of this exercise for those who cannot breathe through either nostril. Practice breathing with only one nostril, inhaling and exhaling, or inhale through the left and exhale by the right nostril several times and then do it in reverse.

Alternate breathing helps calm and steady the mind, cleanses the nasal passages and sinuses, oxygenates and purifies blood, tones and soothes the nerve system, and relaxes and refreshes the body.

Yoga Posture
If you want to get results, you have to follow the process.

In yoga you should do stretching exercises slowly, at your own pace, gradually increasing the amount of movement, bending, and turning in the poses. It is very important to maintain quiet and even breathing—without holding your breath—when you practice yoga postures [3, 16, 20, 21, 22, 24, 29].

Learn to distinguish between normal and unhealthy bodily responses to exercise. *A normal* response includes increased heart rate, more rapid and deep breathing, and minor muscle aches. *Unhealthy* reactions include dizziness, chest pain and shortness of breath, or sudden stabbing pain anywhere.

If you have any back and neck serious conditions, or other medical conditions you are aware of, it is extremely important that you get advice from your doctor to yoga. Additionally, especially if you are new to yoga, it would be most helpful to work with an experienced and knowledgeable yoga teacher to guide you, at least initially.

During yoga practice it is important to pay attention to the rhythmical breathing that will allow you to be aware of the present moment so that you can feel your body's positive sensations. The body usually gives you feedback as to how deeply to go into the posture, what subtle shifts you need to make, and when to come out of the pose.

It is important to pay attention to your breathing because it is a good indicator of control when you begin to feel fatigue, become strained, or have uneven breathing. If you follow your positive sensations and the subtle reactions of your body, you will see how your breath and your body will guide you through yoga practice and through your life.

Choose exercises and postures that are most appropriate to your health condition and your individual physical capability. As a general recommendation in case you have some physical weakness, it would be better to begin practicing yoga postures in lying position. After one or two weeks you can try to do postures sitting on a chair, then after a week or two try to do poses standing against a wall.

When you learn to listen to your body and feel what kind of posture is good for you to do, you will become the best trainer for yourself in improving your health. You will find explanations of each posture with photos below. Yoga stretching is safe for most people and should be done daily, or at least 3-4 times a week. However it is best to do only those postures that give you a sense of comfort. Stop doing any posture if you feel pain or discomfort in any part of your body. Please be especially careful if you have problems with your shoulders, a back injury, or other trauma problems. Those who have osteoporosis should be very gentle doing flexion and extension of the spine, or twisting of the spine. Be aware of your own possibilities and slowly increase the amount of time you hold each posture. Before you start to do yoga postures or warm up exercises, please be prepared and pay attention to recommendations that are important for you. Do the yoga postures with awareness, slowly and carefully without forcing yourself.

If you have some physical limitations that prevent you from practicing yoga postures, you can focus on the breathing exercises, relaxation, and then on meditation. These are accessible to everyone.

Begin practicing yoga postures 1-2 hours before a meal or 3-4 hours after a full meal. Usually our bodies are stiffer in the morning, so it is better to do warm-up exercises in the morning. During evening and nighttime our bodies are more flexible and less stiff, so it is a good time for yoga postures. Practice yoga in a well-ventilated room where there is a source of fresh air, and wear loose clothing.

Here I present three groups of yoga postures with eight or nine stretching exercises in each group: in a lying position on a floor mat, sitting on a chair, and standing against a wall. When you are in a posture, hold it until it is comfortable for your body and then slowly release it. Don't be in a hurry, move your body slowly and consciously. When you hold a pose, focus your mind on slow and rhythmical breathing; relax facial muscles and the muscles around your eyes. Relax your neck and shoulder muscles. The more relaxed you are in any posture, the longer you will be able to hold it. As soon as you feel even the slightest discomfort and tiredness, begin to slowly come out of the pose.

All yoga postures presented in this book are simple, but you will have excellent results if you practice them with awareness. Even warm-up exercises should be done with awareness and with quiet breathing. If you want to receive the highest benefits from healing yoga, you must strive for self-control, self-discipline, and you should practice yoga regularly. Gradually you will be able to practice yoga more easily and you will enjoy it.

Warm-Up Exercises

1. Sitting on a chair, lift up your shoulders and chest as you inhale; hold this position for 2-3 seconds, and then, exhaling, lower your shoulders and relax them. Repeat this exercise 3-5 times. This will help you release tension in your shoulders and chest.

2. As you inhale, roll your shoulders forward and raise them up and then exhaling, roll them back and lower them. Do this exercise several times focusing your attention on your breathing and on the circular movement of your shoulders. Then after a short rest, begin rolling shoulders in reverse: as you inhale, roll your shoulders back and up, and then, exhaling, over and down.

3. Exercises for the neck and head will help you relax your neck and head muscles and make the neck vertebrae more flexible and strong: Sit on a chair with a straight back, inhale slowly, and, then, as you exhale, lower your head onto your chest (Photo 6a). Hold this position and breathe quietly. With each exhalation, allow the muscles of your neck and shoulders to relax more and more, and feel the gentle stretching at the back of your neck. As your neck muscles relax, your head will drop slightly lower and lower. Do not allow your spine to bend with it, keeping the

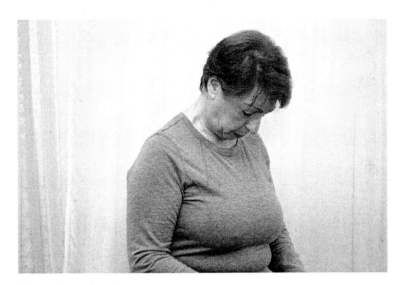

Photo 6a

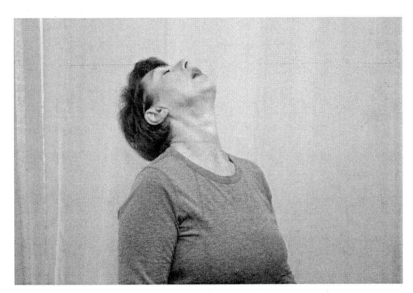

Photo 6b

spine straight continues correct alignment and allows for a deep stretch in the neck muscles. Hold the pose several seconds or as long as it is comfortable for you. Try to be relaxed and keep up rhythmic, diaphragmatic breathing. When you begin to feel even the slightest discomfort, slowly lift your head up as you inhale.

Next, let your head drop gently backwards (Photo 6b), open mouth slightly, hold the pose, and breathe evenly and quietly. Relax your facial muscles and the front of your neck, and relax your shoulders. Hold this pose for several seconds, and then slowly lift your head back to starting position as you inhale. Repeat this exercise 2-3 times.

Next, while keeping your back straight and your shoulders facing forward, swivel your head to the right and hold this position for 2-3 seconds (Photo 6c). Then slowly turn the head to the left. Keep the breathing naturally and rhythmically. It is important to do this movement without tilting your head. Repeat 3-4 times.

Now, with your back straight and your facial muscles and shoulders relaxed, tilt your head toward your right shoulder so that the left side of your neck is gently stretched (Photo 6d). Hold this position for 2-3 seconds and then **slowly** lift your head, rest for one breath, and then lower your head toward your left shoulder. Pay attention to

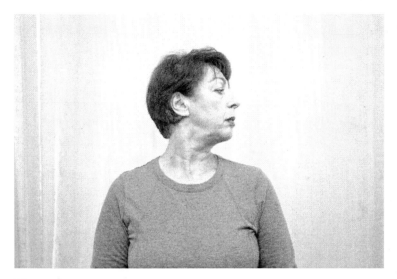

Photo 6c

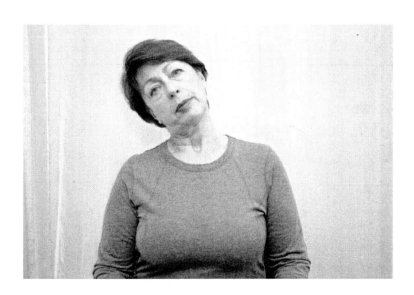

Photo 6d

the gentle stretching in the right side of your neck. Keep up natural rhythmic breathing. Repeat this exercise 2-3 times.

4. This exercise is done in lying position. Keep your knees bent, tighten the muscles of your buttocks and thighs and at the same time draw the lower part of your abdomen in. Hold this tightness for 5-10 seconds, breathe evenly, then release and relax. Repeat 2-3 times. This simple exercise makes the lower part of the spine stronger and strengthens pelvis.

5. Stretching and moving your arms with clasped hands, breathing slowly. Clasp your hands in front of you. As you inhale slowly, stretch your arms downward with palms out (Photo 7a), then, as you exhale, place your palms on your chest (Photo 7b). Hold the pose for several seconds. Next, as you inhale, pull your arms forward with palms out (Photo 8); pauses, then, exhaling, bring your hands back to your chest. Next, taking a deep breath in, stretch your hands up over your head with palm facing out (Photo 9) and after a short pause bring your hands to your chest while you exhale slowly. Next, clasp your hands behind your back, inhale slowly and extend your arms behind your back (Photo 10); then, exhaling, bring your hands to your chest. Then relax. Repeat this cycle 2-3 times.

To strengthen the upper back, raise your arms out to the sides. Bend your elbows; keep them at shoulder level,

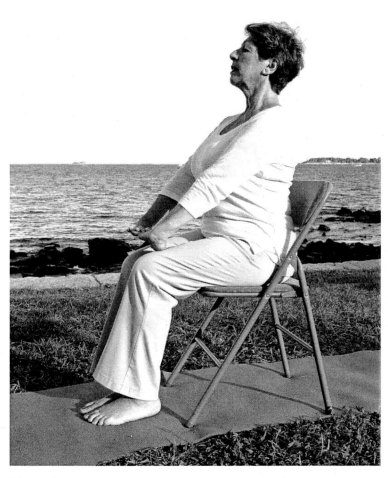

Photo 7a

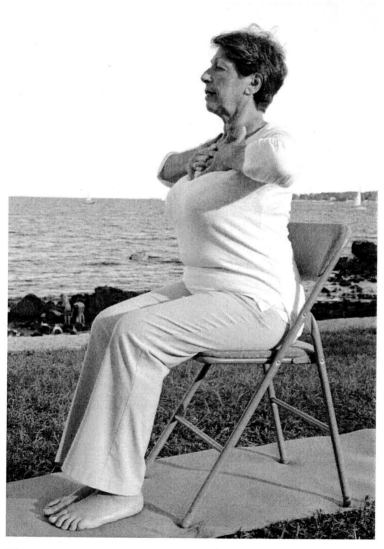

Photo 7b

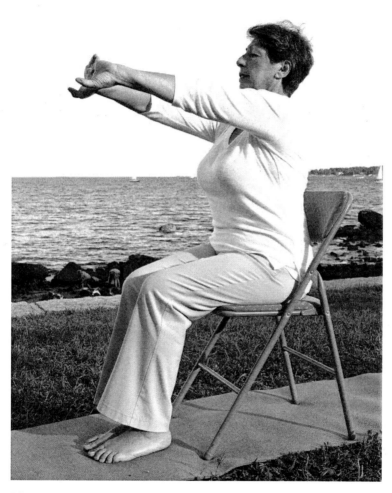

Photo 8

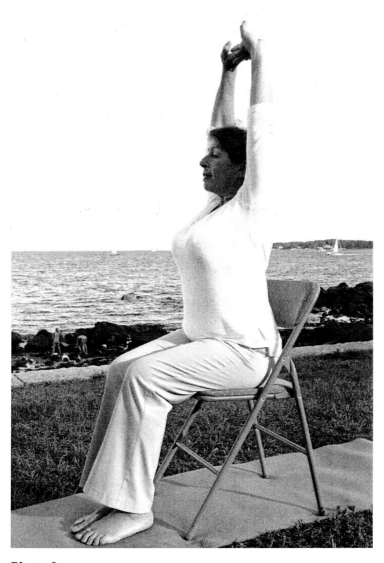

Photo 9

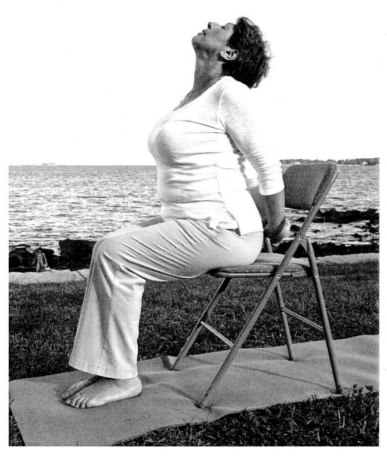

Photo10

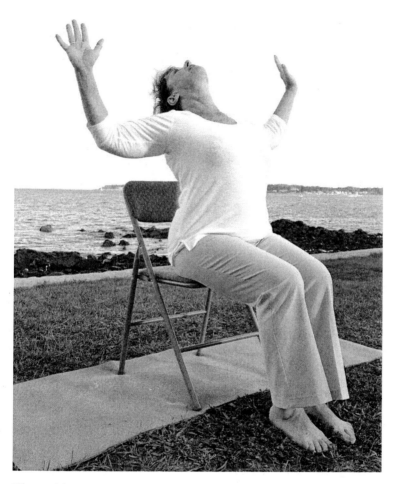

Photo 11

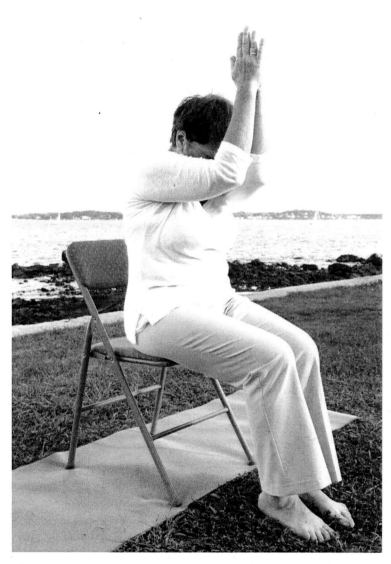

Photo 12

fingers pointing up. As you inhale, move your elbows back while tilting your head backwards; try to move your shoulder blades toward each other (Photo 11). Keep your mouth slightly open. Breathe quietly. Hold the pose for 1-2 seconds. Then as you exhale, move your elbows forward toward your chest (Photo 12). Feel how your shoulder blades stretch as you connect elbows, lower your head to your chest, and hold the pose for 1-3 seconds. Breathe and relax. Repeat 2-5 times.

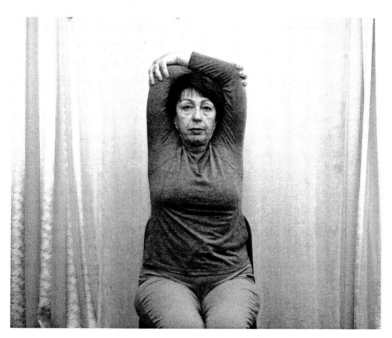

Photo 13

Raise your arms over your head, bend your elbows and grasp them above your head (Photo 13), breathe evenly, keep your back straight and relaxed. Hold the pose for 5-10 seconds.

After doing the Warm-Up Exercises you can practice several yoga postures, or you can rest and do yoga postures later on in the day.

Yoga Postures in Lying Position

When you practice yoga postures in a lying position, it is important to rest, relax and breathe normally between postures.

Lie on your back, inhale slowly and bring your arms up over your head. Your legs and arms should be straight. As you inhale, stretch your feet down, away from your body, while you stretch your arms, up, away from your body. Your toes should be pointed back toward you (Photo 14). Hold this pose 1-3 seconds. Then exhale slowly and relax. Repeat 2-3 times. It is very good to do this pose in the morning to wake your body up.

Lie on your back, bend your knees and bring them up to the abdomen or the chest and hug them with your arms (Photo 15, page 82). Close your eyes, relax your chest, shoulder, neck and facial muscles. Try to keep the back of your shoulders on the floor. If this is difficult for you, use a strap or towel behind your thighs (Photo 16, page 83). Relax your lower back and buttocks. Hold this pose as long as is comfortable for you, but don't force yourself. In the beginning, hold this pose for several seconds and repeat 2-3 times. Eventually you will be able to hold this pose for around a minute.

Benefits: This posture releases tension in the low back and strengthens the abdomen.

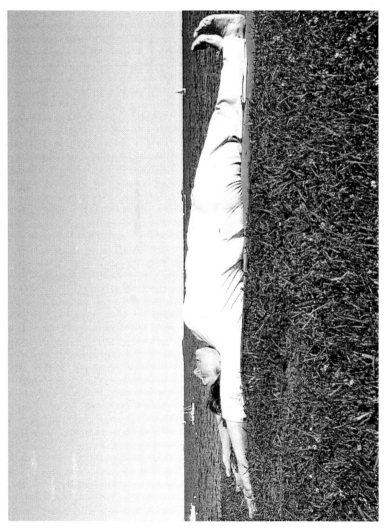

Photo 14

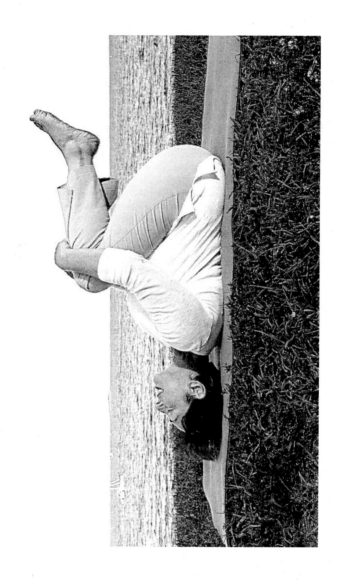

Photo 15

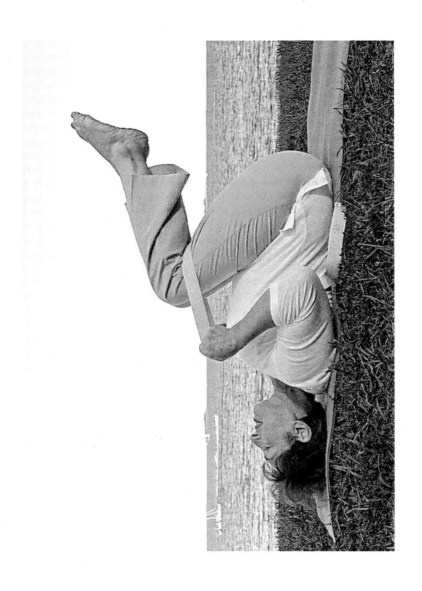

Photo 16

Spinal Twist Posture (Photo 17)

Lie on your back. Bend your knees and press your feet against the floor. Lower your knees toward the floor on the right, and move your torso to the left, while looking toward the left (Photo 17). Breathe evenly and quietly. Gently stretch your knees toward the floor. Extend your arms to the sides at shoulder level and keep your palms up. Hold the pose as long as is comfortable for you, and then at the next inhalation, slowly raise your knees up to starting position and then straighten your legs. Rest, relax your body. And then repeat, lowering your knees to the left side and turning your torso to the right.

Benefits: This spinal twist strengthens the spine and stretches the lower back and outer hips.

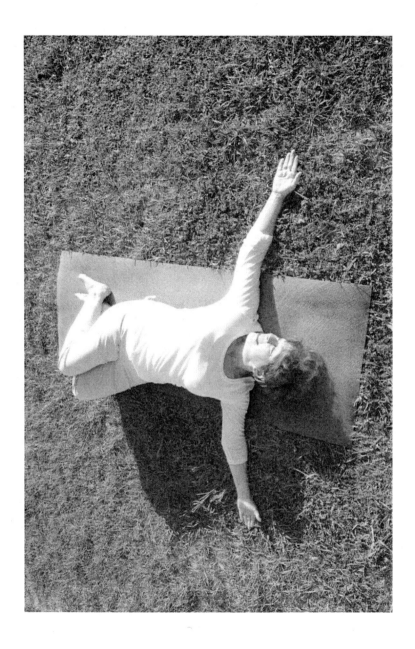

Photo 17

Open Out Twist Posture (Photo 18).

Lie on your stomach. Raise both hands over your head and put them on the floor keeping your arms and legs apart; touch your forehead to the floor. Lift your right arm up and roll your body slightly to the right. Bend your right knee (toward the left) and bring it up onto the floor in front of your body. Keep your left leg straight. Continue to roll your body to the right, and turn your head so that you can see behind you. Relax your facial muscles and shoulders, close your eyes; feel the stretch in your upper and lower body. Breathe and relax. Practice this posture with patience, and gradually you will be able to bring the right arm closer and closer to the floor on the left. Hold this pose as long as is comfortable for you, from 10-30 seconds. Slowly return to the initial pose. Rest in *Crocodile Pose* (see below) before doing the same posture on the other side.

Benefits: This pose is very good for opening your lungs, for expansion of the side ribs, and for stretching the upper and lower back.

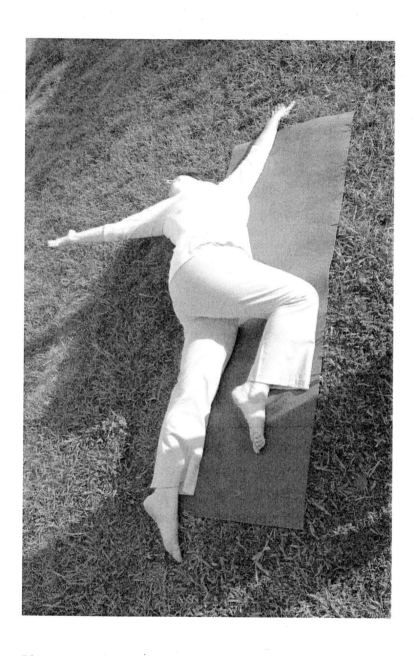

Photo 18

Crocodile Posture (Photo 19)

This is a very good resting pose. Lie face down; keep your feet apart with toes turned out. Lower your forehead onto your forearms. Breathe slowly and deeply, relaxing your body. Hold this pose as long as is comfortable for you.

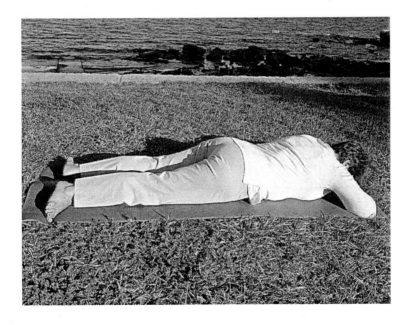

Photo 19

Cobra Posture, easy variation (Photo 20)

Lie on your stomach; lay your forehead on your hands. Quiet your breath and relax. Now with your elbows on the floor, keep the forearms to shoulder level and parallel to each other. In this pose the spine is gently bent toward the back. Press your navel against the floor. Breathe quietly and evenly. Keep your feet together. Relax your upper body and concentrate on feeling the stretch between the shoulder blades. Close your eyes, mentally look up, and relax your facial muscles, neck and shoulders. Try to keep your head, neck and chest aligned with one another. In the beginning, hold the pose for several seconds and then slowly release it, bringing your head down to your hands. Repeat 2-3 times. Gradually you will be able to hold this pose longer, from 20-60 seconds.

Benefits: This posture strengthens the back, especially the upper back, stretches the chest, and improves your posture.

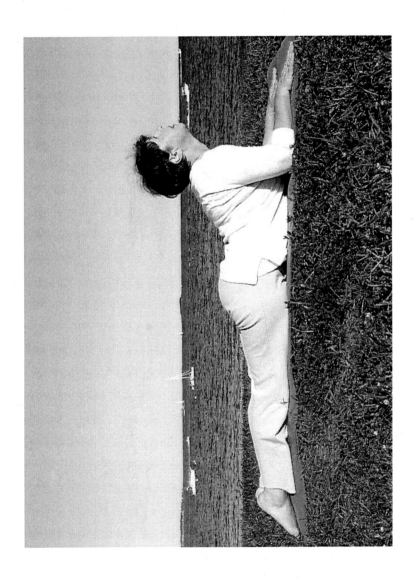

Photo 20

98

Cat Posture (Photos 21, 22)

Stand on your knees and put your palms on the floor. Keep your hands on the floor at shoulder width, fingers pointed forward. Keep your knees slightly apart. Your thighs and arms are vertical. Your back is parallel to the floor.

The Cat Posture has two parts. In the first part (Photo 21) drop the middle of the back as you inhale. Let it lower down while you lift your head up. Your mouth is slightly open. Focus your mind on the middle of your back, keeping your arms straight. Breathe evenly. Hold this pose for 3-5 seconds. Then move smoothly and slowly into the second part of the posture (Photo 22). As you breathe out, arch the middle of your spine as high as you can and lower your head down between your arms. Continue diaphragmatic breathing and hold this pose several seconds. With each exhalation pull your abdominal muscles in, towards the spine. Repeat this pose several times.

Benefits: This posture increases flexibility in your back, tones the nervous system, and improves circulation.

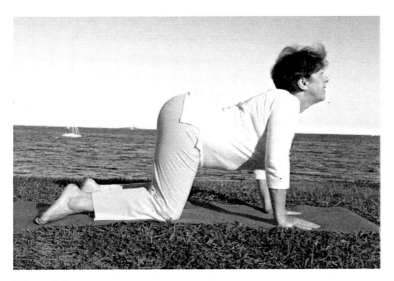

Photo 21

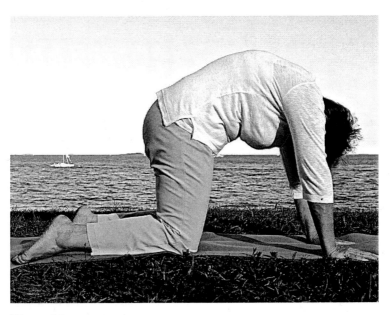

Photo 22

Star Posture (Photos 23, 24)

Sit down on the floor. Cross your legs and extend the knees out to the side. Bring the soles of your feet together and clasp your feet with your hands. Place your feet at a point on the floor that feels comfortable, stretching your knees out to the sides as much as you can. Do not force yourself. Breathe evenly. Relax facial muscles, neck and shoulders. Then take a deep breath and while exhaling, lean forward as long as you feel comfortable, keeping your back straight. Then lower your head onto your chest without feeling discomfort (Photo 23).

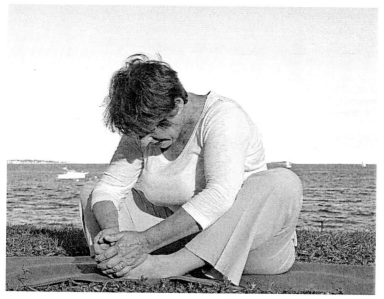

Photo 23

Hold your feet with your hands gently pressing your forearms into your calves, slowly moving your knees down to the floor. Hold this pose for 5-6 seconds. Gradually, with practice, hold the pose for 10-15 seconds. Then, inhaling, slowly raise your head, your chest and then your back. Rest and repeat one more time.

You can simplify this pose, by crossing your legs and keeping your feet turned inward (Photo 24). Try to keep your back straight, and hold this pose for several seconds.

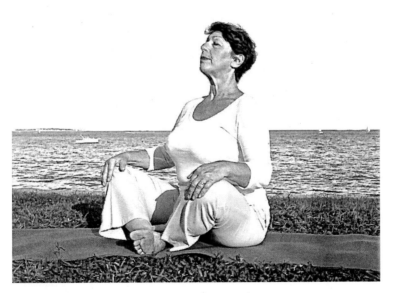

Photo 24

Put your hands on your knees and gently press them down to the floor. You may feel some slight tension in the knees, hips and ankles. Do not overstretch. Release, stretch your legs and rest. Repeat this pose crossing your legs in the opposite direction, i.e. move the foot that was inside to the outside. It is good to do this pose every day.

Benefits: This posture pulls on and opens the pelvis, limbers up the spine, strengthens the hips, lower back and legs, and improves digestion.

Bridge Posture (Photo 25)

It is good to do this pose after the *Star Pose.* Lie on the floor on your back, bend your knees, keeping them slightly apart and pressing your feet to the floor. Keep your arms beside your body. Lift your buttocks off the floor by a few inches. Keep your thighs and the inner sides of your feet parallel. Feel that your feet and shoulder blades are pressed against the floor. Breathe from your diaphragm quietly and rhythmically. Relax your buttocks. Relax your facial muscles and neck. Slightly arch your lower vertebrae. The more relaxed you are the longer you will be able to stay in the pose. At the beginning, hold the pose several seconds, and then as you exhale, release, slowly bringing your spine down onto the floor. Repeat this pose one more time.

Benefits: This pose stretches the chest, neck, abdomen, and the front of the thighs; it also strengthens the back and stimulates the abdominal organs and lungs.

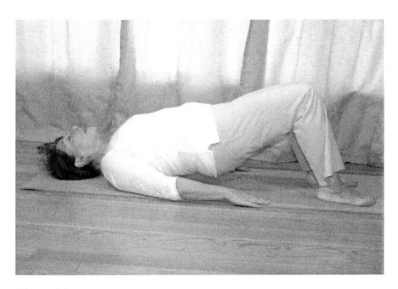

Photo 25

Yoga Postures while Sitting on a Chair

The Mountain Pose (Photos 26, 27)

Sit on a chair. Relax your abdominal muscles, feel them soften, and keep your back straight. As you inhale, raise your arms over your head and fold your hands together. The hands in this posture form the peak of a mountain. The fingers should be pointing upward. Hold your chest, neck and head up in one line. Take 2-3 slow, deep breaths while holding this pose, and with each inhalation stretch your hands a little higher, but only if it is possible for you. In the beginning, keep your elbows bent at shoulder level (Photo 26). Hold the pose for 5-15 seconds, and then, slowly exhaling, release, lower your arms and relax. By practicing this pose you will eventually be able to stretch your arms straight and hold them closer to your ears (Photo 27).

Benefits: This pose improves your posture and balance, increases flexibility of the spine, and increases circulation in the lungs.

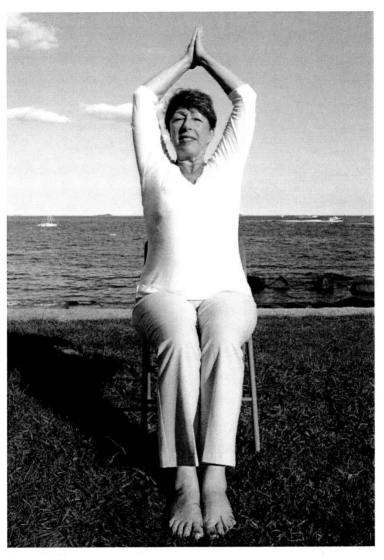

Photo 26

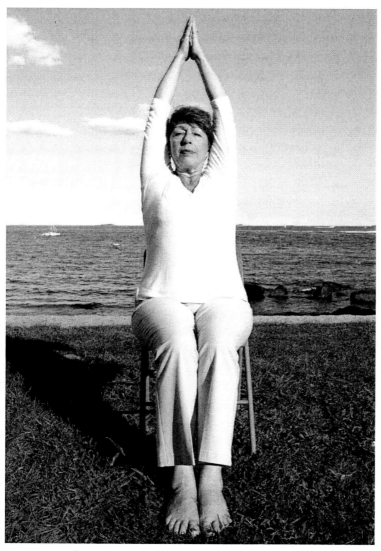

Photo 27

The Cat Posture Sitting in a Chair (Photos 28, 29)

Sit in the middle of the chair. Extend your legs wide, press your hands onto your knees. Move your body slightly forward, and then while inhaling, arch the middle of your back tilting your head backward. Keep your mouth slightly open. Concentrate on the middle point of your back (Photo 28). Hold the pose several for seconds while breathing normally. On the exhalation, release and curve your back. Move slowly your head onto your chest. Hold this pose for several seconds, breathing evenly (Photo 29). Concentrate your mind on the center of your spine and stretch it. Repeat 3-5 times.

Benefits: This pose helps increase flexibility in your spine. When practiced regularly, this pose can help decrease back pain. It also stretches your neck and helps to stimulate your abdominal organs.

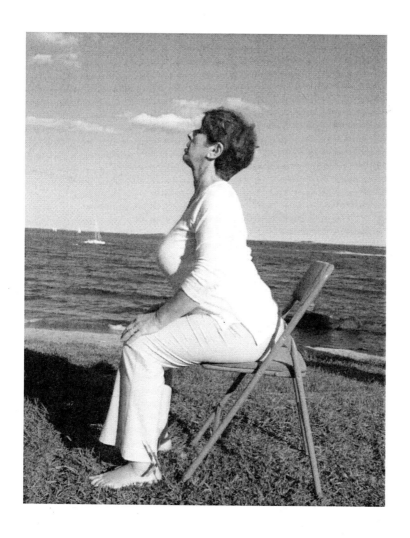

Photo 28

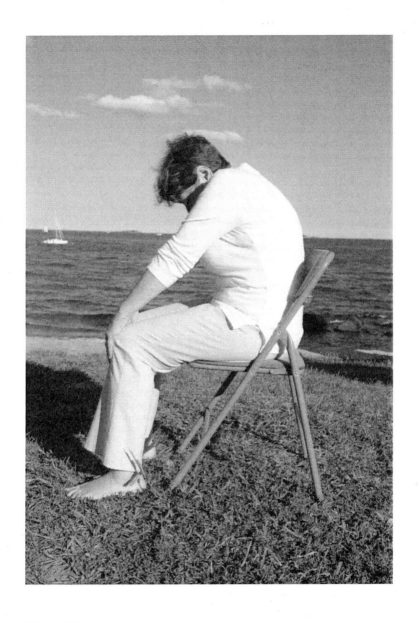

Photo 29

Forward Bend Posture (Photo 30)

Sit on a chair, spread your legs wide. Inhaling, raise your hands up while straightening the spine and then as you exhale, slowly bend forward, relaxing your back, neck and head, feeling all your muscles releasing. Allow your arms and shoulders to hang freely (Photo 30) or feel to only go into forward bends to 90 degrees, with hands on the thighs. Relax your facial muscles. Breathe quietly and evenly, and with each exhalation, continue to progressively relax the muscles of your back, head and shoulders. Be super gentle – even image the posture of the neck, rather than doing it all the way. Breathe slowly and deeply, and with each exhalation feel your torso lengthen effortlessly. Hold the pose 10-15 seconds or as long as is comfortable for you. Then, as you inhale, slowly come up from the pose. Repeat 2-3 times. If you have high blood pressure, avoid this pose. You can try to do a *Modified Forward Bend* (Page 105).

Benefits: This pose releases tension in the neck and shoulders and stretches your lower back and torso.

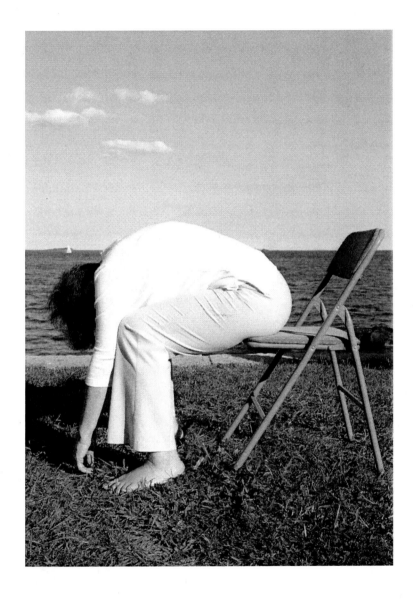

Photo 30

Modified Forward Bend (Photo 31)

Sit down on a blanket with your legs wide apart. Place your chair in front of you far enough away so that you can place your forehead on the chair seat. You can place a folded blanket under your forehead for comfort. Slightly bend your back forward. Bring your arms over your head and put them on the sides of the chair, finding the most comfortable position for them. Breathe evenly. Relax your body, especially your facial muscles, upper back and neck. Breathe and relax. Hold this pose as long as it is easy for you. Then inhale and slowly come out of the pose.

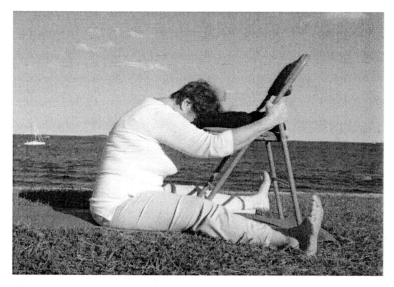

Photo 31

Backbend Posture (Photos 32, 33)

Sit on a full chair seat, the back of the chair should be on the level of your shoulders. As you inhale, lift up your arms and lean back over the back of the chair. Reach your arms up and back. Tilt your head back, keeping your mouth open, and relax your jaw. Feel your spine stretching (Photo 32). Breathe and relax. Hold this pose for several seconds, and then as you inhale slowly come up and release.

If this pose is difficult for you, try doing the easy variant (Photo 33). Sit in the middle of the chair seat. Clasp your hands behind your back. Stretch your arms away from you while tilting your head back. Keep your mouth slightly open and relax your facial muscles. Breathe evenly. Hold the pose for 3-5 seconds. Slowly come back from this position on the exhale.

Benefits: This pose helps limber the lower and upper back.

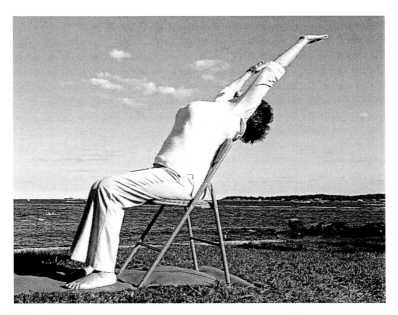

Photo 32

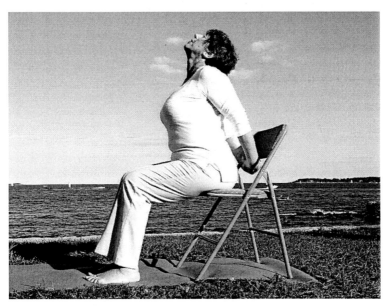

Photo 33

Seated Spinal Twist (Photo 34)

Sit in the middle of a chair seat, and then turn your body, legs and feet to the right so that the back of the chair is to your right. Position your feet, knees and hips a little apart. Inhale slowly and raise your arms up overhead, then as you exhale, turn your upper body to the right. Place your hands on the back of the chair. Turn your head and look to the right. Keep the spine straight. Breathe slowly and deeply. Relax your facial muscles and shoulders. As you relax into the pose, try to twist your spine a little further. Hold the pose a few seconds or longer if you feel comfortable. Breathe and relax. Slowly release and come back to the initial pose. Rest and repeat the pose on the opposite side.

Benefits: This pose increases circulation and flexibility in the spine and hips.

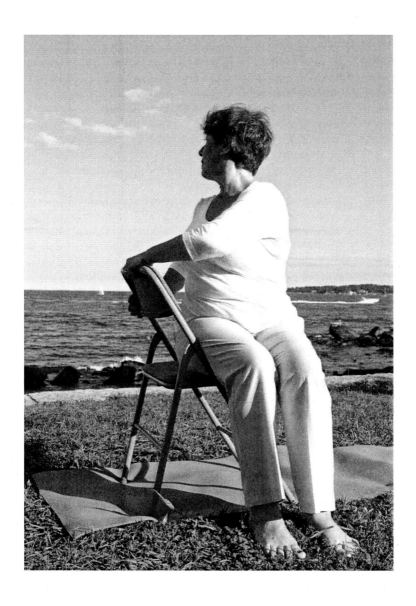

Photo 34

Side Stretch Posture (Photo 35)

Sit on a chair with a straight spine and without leaning against the back of the chair. Hold on to the right side of the chair, keeping your right elbow bent. As you inhale, slowly raise and stretch the left arm up, and, then, while exhaling, bend your body to the right. Feel the stretch in the left side of your body. Don't lean forward. Breathe evenly. Drop your head gently to the right shoulder; relax your facial muscles and shoulders. Hold the pose as long as you feel comfortable. On the inhalation, slowly come out of the pose. Rest, and then repeat bending to the left side. You can do this posture 2-3 times.

Benefits: This poses releases back tension and increases flexibility of the sides.

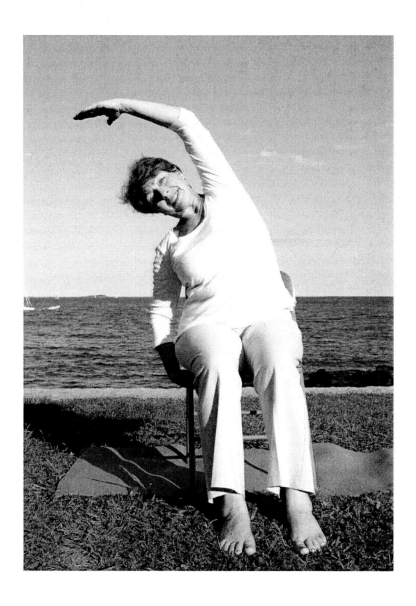

Photo 35

Seated Half Lotus (Photo 36)

Sit on a chair. Lift your right leg, grasp it with your hands and place the right foot on the left knee so that your right sole is facing up. Put your hands on the crease of your hips, elbows pointed back. Inhale deeply, and then exhaling, slowly lean forward while tilting your head slightly forward. Relax your facial muscles and neck, and also relax your chest and belly. Feel a balance between intensity and softness. Do not push yourself too much. Keep your spine extended. Breathe quietly and rhythmically. When you begin to feel tired, sit up and slowly bring your right foot to the floor. Rest, relaxing your breathing and then repeat this pose with the left leg.

Benefits: This pose stretches your hips and buttocks; it is also very good for the flexibility of your knees.

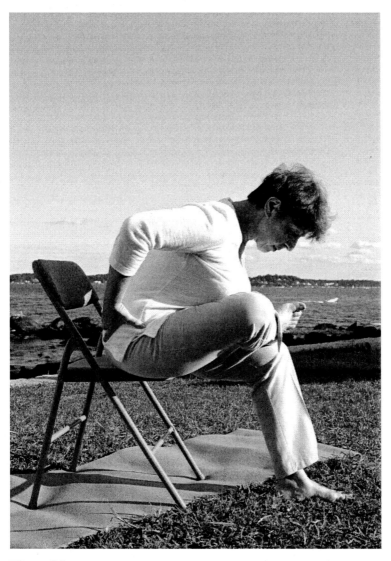

Photo 36

Seated Cobra Pose (Photo 37)

Sit in the middle of the chair seat. Raise your arms over your head, bend your elbows and grasp them above your head. Keep your elbows wide. As you inhale, feel the expansion of your ribcage. Relax your facial muscles and jaw. Continue breathing rhythmically and draw your abdomen in, closer to the spine. Arch the upper back. Feel as if your chest were open and stretched. Focus your mind on the point between your shoulder blades. Hold this pose as long as it is comfortable for you. Do not overdo it. Then as you exhale, slowly release your arms; rest with some quiet breathing. If you hold this pose for only 3-5 seconds, you can repeat it one more time. With practice you will be able to hold the pose about 20-30 seconds, and you will be getting the most benefit from it.

Benefits: This pose open the chest, strengthens the back, stretches the ribcage, and improves your lungs.

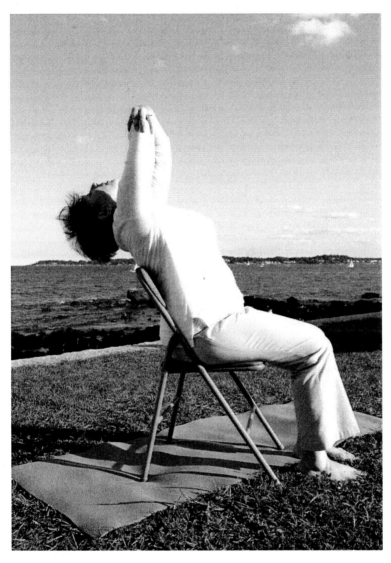

Photo 37

Yoga Postures Standing Near the Wall

Stand with your back against the wall. Straighten your spine and your entire body from head to toe. Press the back of your head, shoulder blades, and buttocks against the wall. Breathe naturally and relax your whole body. Keep your head, neck, and chest aligned with each other. To intensify this pose, raise your arms to the sides, press them against the wall, and hold them at shoulder level. Hold this pose a few seconds or as long as is comfortable for you, and then release it and rest. You can do this pose several times a day to maintain right posture.

Mountain Posture (Photo 38a, 38b)

Stand with your back against the wall. Keep your feet together. Tense your muscles from the toes up to the waist, hold this tension, and at the same time relax the upper body from the waist up, especially your shoulders, chest, neck, and facial muscles. Breathe slowly and deeply. As you inhale, raise your arms over your head, keep your palms together and slightly bend your elbows (Photo 38a). The hands in this posture form the peak of a mountain. The fingers should be pointing upward. Keep your chest, neck

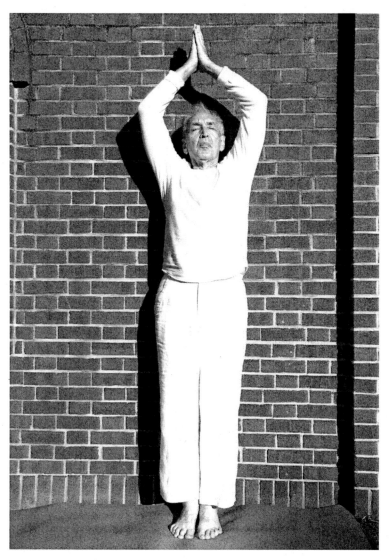

Photo 38a

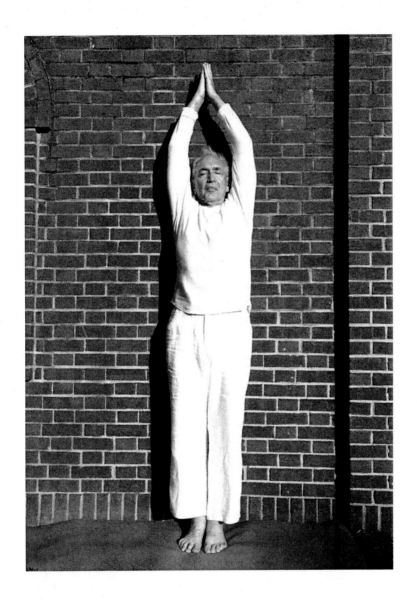

Photo 38b

and head aligned. With each inhalation, stretch your arms as far up as is possible for you. With practice you will be able to straighten your arms and slightly press your forearms to your ears (Photo 38b). Hold this pose from 5-10 seconds or a little longer if you feel comfortable. Then exhaling, slowly lower your arms and relax. Repeat this pose once or twice more.

Benefits: This pose supports muscular and skeletal alignment, strengthens the upper back and lungs.

Right Angle Posture (Photos 39, 40)

Stand a few steps away from a wall, facing it. Bend your knees a little and then bend forward slightly from the top of your thighs, and move your hips back until your torso is parallel to the floor. Put your hands on the wall and try to keep your arms parallel to the floor (39). Lengthen your spine, putting the pressure of your weight onto your legs. Continue rhythmical, abdominal breathing. Keep your back, neck and head aligned. As you exhale, draw your abdominal muscles toward your spine, so you feel your abdomen tighter which creates a stretch in your lower back.

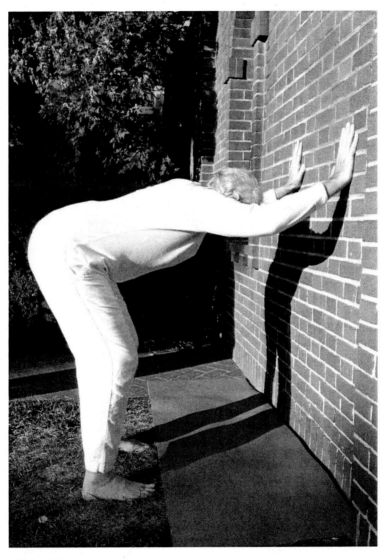

Photo 39

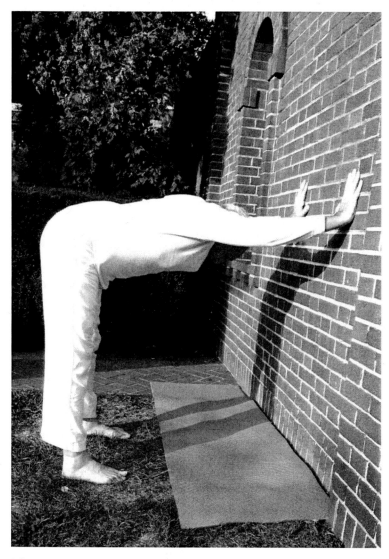

Photo 40

Hold this pose for several seconds or as long as is comfortable for you, and then slowly release it.

With practice you will be able to intensify this pose (Photo 40). Put your hands a little down the wall, in line with your hips, so that your torso becomes a right angle to your legs. Press your hands more intensely against the wall. Keep your legs straight. Breathe and relax. Hold the pose several seconds or as long as is comfortable for you.

Benefits: This pose releases tension in your back, and stretches your hamstrings, calves, chest and back. It is especially good to do the pose after you have been sitting or lying for a long time.

Warrior Posture I (Photo 41)

This is a strengthening pose. Stand in *Mountain Posture* (Photo 38) with your back leaning against the wall. Place your feet wide apart, as far as is comfortably possible. Turn to the right so that your right foot is turned 90 degrees, and your left foot is turned to about a 45 degrees angle. The knee on the turned your foot should not exceed the toes so that the knee joint stays properly supported. To feel more balanced, lean with the right side of your body, the right hip and shoulder against the wall. Now as you exhale, bend your right knee until your thigh is parallel to the floor or as close as is comfortable for you. Do not bend your left knee and hold your left leg straight. Raise your arms overhead; join the palms of your hands together. Breathe slowly and deeply. To complete this pose, bring your head back and gaze up at your hands. Slightly open your mouth and relax your face. Hold the pose for 5-10 seconds, and then slowly lower your arms, straighten your knees and place your feet together as in *Mountain Pose*. Rest, relax, and repeat the pose on the left side.

Benefits: This pose strengthens ankles, knees, hips, and spine; expands the chest; improves balance and concentration; and improves your mood. Yogic wisdom informs us that this and the few next postures also increase self-confidence.

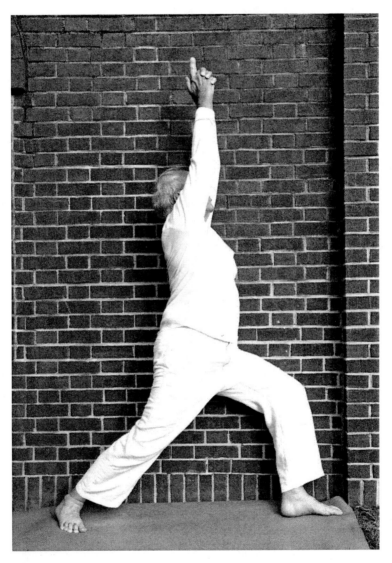

Photo 41

Warrior Posture II (Photo 42)

Begin the pose the same as in Warrior I. Lean your back and buttocks against the wall. Stand upright with feet spread wide apart, turn your right foot to 90 degrees, and the left to 45 degrees, and raise your arms out at shoulder level; keep the arms parallel to the floor, palms down. Now as you exhale, bend your right knee until your thigh is parallel to the floor or as close as is comfortable for you. Do not force yourself. The left leg is straight. Turn your head to the right and gaze at the fingers of your right hand. Keep your head, neck and chest aligned and pressed to the wall. Relax your facial muscles and neck. Hold the pose for not more than 10 seconds. Then slowly lower your arms and place your feet together. Rest, relax, and repeat the pose on the left side.

Benefits: The pose is intensified from Warrior I.

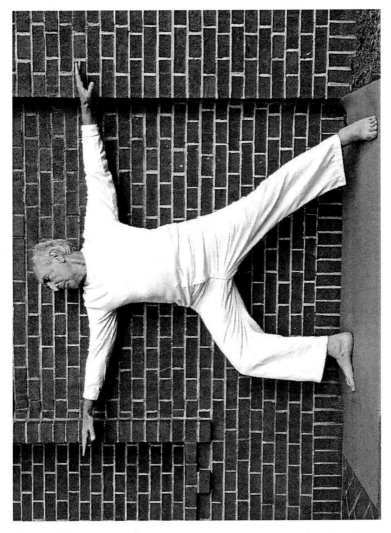

Photo 42

Triangle Posture (Photo 43)

This pose is very beneficial but requires practice before you will be able to do it correctly. In the beginning try to perform the pose as best you can and do not force yourself.

Stand with your back leaning against the wall and place your feet wide apart. Turn your right foot parallel to the wall at 90 degrees; turn your left foot approximately 45 degrees. Take a deep breath in and extend your arms out to the sides at shoulder level. Now bend to the right from the waist; place your right hand at a comfortable point on the right leg—on the knee, the calf, or the ankle. The left arm is stretched up and back. With practice you will be able to keep your arms and legs straight. Turn your head and look up at the upraised hand. Try to stretch your spine slowly, and bring your torso and head in line with your right leg. Continue the rhythmical, abdominal breathing. Hold the pose for 5-10 seconds, and then slowly return to the initial pose, releasing your arms and bringing your feet together. Rest, relax, and repeat the pose on the left side.

Benefits: This pose firms and tones the leg muscles, expands the chest and improves lung functions, and strengthens the back and abdomen.

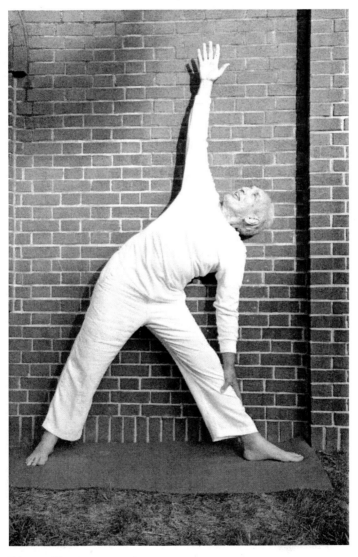

Photo 43

Forward Bend Posture (Photo 44)

Stand with your back against the wall. Place your feet slightly apart and one step away from the wall. Move your hips back so that your buttocks press against the wall. Lean forward, keeping your spine straight. If you need to, bend your knees so that you can lengthen your spine. Grasp your elbows with your hands. Let your head and arms drop down feeling the stretch in your back and neck. Continue your abdominal, rhythmical breathing. Relax your facial muscles, neck and shoulders. Imagine your body is heavy, soft and relaxed. Hold the pose for 10-15 seconds or longer, until you feel uncomfortable. On exhaling release your arms, slowly come up and rest. You can repeat the pose one more time.

Benefits: This pose stretches the hamstrings, calves, and back. It also releases tension in the shoulders and back.

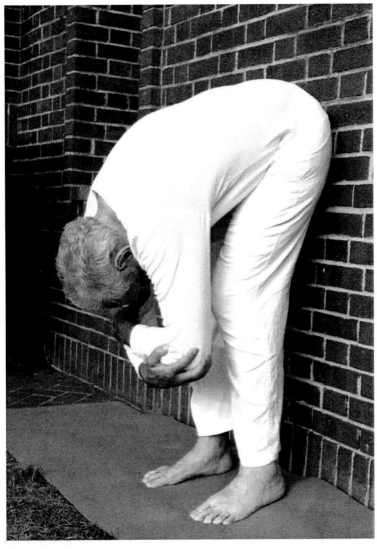

Photo 44

Backward Bending Posture (Photo 45)

Stand with your back a step or two away from the wall. Keep your feet slightly apart. As you inhale, raise your arms over your head and take 2-3 deep, slow breaths. Then with next exhalation, bend backward until your hands touch the wall. Slightly bend your knees, if you need to, and tilt your head back. Relax your facial muscles and neck. Breathe and relax. You will feel an expansion in your chest and ribcage. Hold this pose for 2-5 seconds or longer as it is comfortable for you. The moment you feel tired release the pose as you exhale, rest, and repeat it one more time.

Benefits: This pose opens the chest, strengthens the back.

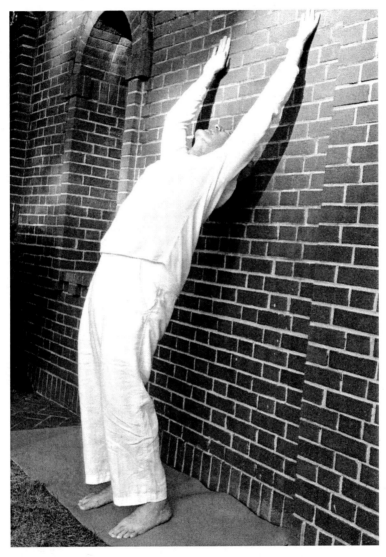

Photo 45

Spinal Twist Posture (Photo 46)

Stand with your feet a small step away from the wall but with your back leaning against the wall. Keep your feet several inches away from each other. Keep your back straight and relaxed. Take a deep breath, and then exhale slowly while turning your upper body toward the right, into a spinal twist. Press your palms against the wall; this will help you deepen the twist. If you have pain in the back do only the gentle spinal twist keeping two bend knees together.

Focus your mind on the middle of your back and feel your spinal column straighten, turn your head to the right, and keep your head, neck and chest aligned with each other. Relax your facial muscles and breathe evenly and quietly. Hold this pose for several seconds or as long as is comfortable for you. With your next exhalation slowly release your twist. Rest and repeat this pose on the left side.

Benefits: The pose releases back tension, and makes your back more flexible.

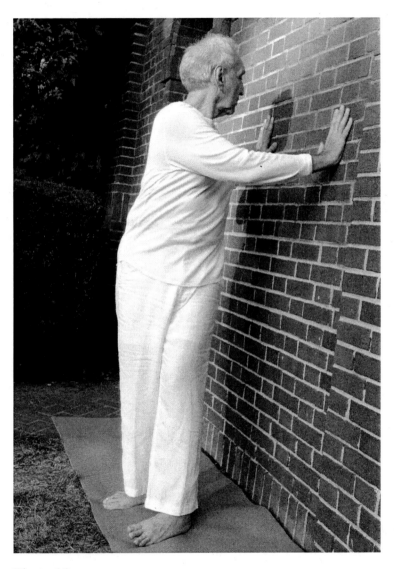

Photo 46

Relaxation

Relaxation is the most important element in the yoga system. It can also be the most difficult posture to maintain. Sometimes people are sitting on the couch in a comfortable position, having a good rest at the end of a stressful day and they think that they are relaxed. But this "comfortable" pose does little to reduce tiredness and stress. In any resting pose, even when you sleep, some muscles continue to be tensed. Yoga teaches us to practice deep relaxation after doing stretching, postures and breathing exercises. It allows us to bring awareness to the full release of muscle tension in deep relaxation [3, 24, 26, and 27]. Conscious relaxation, practiced with calm breathing, also helps bring peace to the mind and energy into balance. Relaxation should be done in a lying or sitting position. In the beginning, do relaxation while lying on your back on a floor mat. In this position it is easiest to maintain diaphragmatic breathing and let muscle tension go. After practicing for some period of time, you will also be able to be relaxed in a sitting position.

Regular breathing exercises really help to progress your relaxation practice. When you inhale and exhale smoothly and rhythmically, you teach your mind to have control over feelings of panic and anxiety. By learning to breathe correctly you are also learning to keep a racing heart or shortness of breath under control. For people suffering from panic, the practice of yoga breathing and relaxation are most effective as a self-healing method.

Learn to guide yourself in relaxation by your inner voice. To do this, read the instructions aloud 2-3 times, and then record yourself reading the instructions. Speak quietly and allow short pauses between instructions. Gradually, with practice, you will be able to do these guided relaxations mentally, listening to your inner voice instead of the recording. You can also ask somebody to help you by recording the relaxation instructions. But it is much better to guide yourself with your own voice, and in a few weeks of self-training you will feel pleased to be able to listen to your inner voice and be guided by yourself.

Beginning of relaxation. Lie on the floor and for the first 2-4 minutes just mentally observe your body. When you are lying on your back, keep your legs a little apart, toes pointed away; your arms should be alongside your body, with palms open. If you sit in a chair, keep your palms open on your knees and your feet slightly apart.

Close your eyes. Concentrate on your breath and quiet it. Concentrate your mind on your navel and notice how it moves up and down as you inhale and exhale. Relax your breathing, holding it for a very short moment after each exhalation. Now bring your attention to your feet and let them go ... Relax your toes ... ankles ... calves ... knees ... and hips. Feel your muscles becoming soft and all tension letting go. Now notice your legs... and let them relax. Feel your legs and feet completely relaxed. Now focus on your arms and hands. Relax your fingers and palms... forearms ... and upper arms ... Bring attention to your arms and hands and then feel them relaxed. Now let go of any tension in your buttocks ... lower back ... muscles of the whole spine ... Feel the back muscles soften. Relax your shoulder blades ... Relax your shoulders. Now mentally watch your abdominal muscles, let the tension go, feel your belly soften ... Now relax your chest ... and relax your ribcage muscles ... notice your body, breathe calmly and rhythmically. Feel that your body is relaxed and you are letting go. Now relax your neck ... feel the back of your neck relaxed ... the front of your neck ... the left side ... and the right side. Now relax your face, relax your chin ... tongue ... lips ... cheeks... eyes and eyelids ... eyebrows and forehead. Mentally look at your face and feel the facial muscles softening and letting go. And now relax your head and scalp ... Feel your body deeply relaxed and be aware of it. Feel your breathing quiet and rhythmical.

Relax your emotions... relax your mind ... feel each muscle of your body deeply relaxed ... aware of the deep peace within and around you. And now with each exhalation, mentally say to yourself with short pauses: "I am relaxed ... relaxed ... relaxed ... I am calm ... I am calm ... I am calm ... I am at peace... I am at peace... I am at peace..."

Go within and enjoy this sense of deep relaxation, deep peace and calmness. In 10-15 minutes, or when you feel that you are ready to come out from relaxation, move your toes and fingers, gently turn your head to each side, take two deep, slow breaths. And then on an inhalation, raise your hands above your head, stretching them. Tense all the muscles in your body, and, exhaling, lower your arms back down alongside your body. Repeat 2-3 times. *of Relaxation is ended.* And then think of how you felt before and how you feel now after relaxation. Notice the difference. Are you calmer? Do you have more energy? Are you more peaceful? Do you feel an energy balance? If your answers are "Yes" it means that you were deeply relaxed and received the full benefit.

To improve and deepen your relaxation practice, view the sources listed at the end of the book.

Strength of Mind and Affirmations

"Be a master of mind rather than mastered by mind."

Zen Saying

To decrease muscle tension, you can learn relaxation rather quickly. But to relax and calm your mind and emotions may take more time. Yoga helps us learn to create the right attitude and develop positive thoughts, to accept circumstances as they are, to realize that perhaps we cannot change stressful situations but we can change ourselves. Spiritual yoga shows us that it is important to realize and be aware that love, peace, joy, and calmness are within us, and we can open these feelings in ourselves, rejecting negative emotions and mental tension [1, 7, 8, 12, 17, and 29].

Developing positive thoughts

We live in two worlds at the same time, or in two realities: the inner reality of our thoughts, feelings and attitudes; and the outer world where there are people, our relationships with them, jobs, places, things and events. Our inner world is sensitive. The mind usually reacts to outside stimuli, but, as yogic wisdom tells us, each of us has a tremendous amount of life force or subtle energy that can be opened and used for self-healing and self-protection. People usually want to change somebody or something in the outer world but, as yoga teaches, it is more important to learn how to develop from within—improving our inner visual image of ourselves, learning how to be free from fear, how to improve mood, and making our attitudes positive. This helps us understand and accept situations in the outer world and improve our perception of the world around us. Spiritual yoga shows us that we should develop the ability to defend ourselves from negative feelings caused by stress.

Great potential energy saved up within the nerve cells of our central nervous system is often blocked by mental tension, by negative thoughts and negative emotions such as anxiety, worry, anger and doubts. Every thought is a vibration of energy in the brain cells, and at the same time it stems from the working of the brain. I mentioned above the connection between mind and body, and how the body and soul easily "hear" thoughts of the mind.

A single thought is not very powerful; it comes and goes. But repeated many times it becomes more focused, directed, and strong. For instance, you have a magnifying glass through which the sunrays pass. If you move it from side to side, the energy of sunlight is dispersed and it does not reveal the strength of the sun's rays. But when you hold the glass still, the concentration of the sun's rays gets so strong that it can cause a fire.

Yoga mental exercises for improving concentration and potential strength

Yoga teachings explain that everyone can practice specific mental exercises to improve concentration and to learn how a focused thought increases its potential strength. It seems that it is easy for us to be a prisoner of our dreams, worries, desires, and negative thoughts, such as: *"I cannot do this," "I am afraid to fail," "I'm not ready,"* and *"I'm too tired."* Practicing mind concentration is very important in achieving a positive direction for our thoughts and to control them. Unfortunately our minds are not accustomed to discipline, so in the beginning, mental exercises and attempts to concentrate may not be so successful, but it is possible to achieve success by using determination, time and repetition. So do not be disappointed if you fail in the first few days of practice. Try to be patient with yourself and you will develop these new skills.

With age, concentration is often diminished but not lost. The most important type of concentration is that which helps you to be aware of the present moment and to pay more attention to what you are doing in the moment, and to your thoughts—in other words, presence. The easiest exercise is simply thinking about yourself in the present moment, where you are right now, notice how and where you are sitting or standing, what you hear, what you see around you. Focus on your emotions, what you feel at this moment, what your attitude is toward the people or things around you, what you like or dislike; pay attention to your breathing, be aware of this moment of your life—all these are very helpful for strengthening your mind and improving your concentration. Do these exercises at least once a day.

Visualization and self-confidence

Another good exercise is to visualize a situation that has not yet happened. Be still and imagine somebody you might meet, or imagine yourself in a certain situation and the reactions would you have. What would you talk about, how would you answer the expected questions, and how would you resolve any forthcoming difficulties? Such practice may help protect you, and allow you to be calmer and emotionally stronger when you are facing life's problems.

Suppose you want to develop self-confidence. Imagine yourself as a confident person. Visualize yourself acting fearlessly while talking with people. Imagine a certain situation that is generally causing you worries, and visualize yourself overcoming those problems. Imagine that you are proud of yourself; imagine the satisfaction and self-confidence you would feel; and imagine how your self-confidence would improve the situation.

People are constantly creating mental images, and if these images are positive, they are filled with positive energy and they become a source of change. Positive mental pictures become a real positive power that works for you. Any thought that comes to mind and then is reinforced has an impact on your life.

In the words of Mahatma Gandhi:

Your beliefs become your thoughts,
Your thoughts become your words,
Your words become your actions,
Your actions become your habits,
Your habits become your values,
Your values become your destiny.

Affirmations and positive mental attitudes

What helps create a positive mental attitude? It is never too late to start helping yourself and to begin to develop strength of mind. In yoga, positive self-suggestions or affirmations are considered the easiest method for developing positive thinking and feeling. This method has been used for centuries in religion, magic and in spiritual systems in the form of prayers and mantras. Affirmations are just words, but with deep meaning—and a person can repeat them aloud or silently. You can do it everywhere: in the doctor's waiting room, in the kitchen, in bed before going to sleep, while driving, walking. But the best time is when you sit quietly repeating affirmation attentively thinking about their content. If you find yourself in an uncomfortable situation you can repeat to yourself some affirmation like, *"I am calm and relaxed, I am calm and relaxed."* Do not force yourself to calm down and relax, just keep repeating these positive statements and watch how your body and emotions obey your inner voice and these positive thoughts.

Believe in the power of positive affirmations because they affect your mind and influence the development of positive attitudes, thoughts and feelings. The human brain can hold only one thought in each moment, so positive affirmations fill the brain, reinforcing your effort to reach your goal at that moment. The mind is the creative force of the brain, so words fill the brain with a predisposition towards what kind of thoughts should be created. As yogic wisdom tells us, to be successful, affirmations should be repeated not less than five times—so it is recommended that we repeat affirmations loudly, then a little more softly, then a whisper, and then just mentally repeat the affirmations two or three times. Yoga teaches that only the fifth repetition goes into the subconscious and helps maintain a positive attitude.

It is not necessary to believe in what you try to affirm. But if you do believe, its impact is much greater. Not believing isn't harmful though, because the brain's function is to choose the content of your thoughts. You do not need to make a special effort. Affirmations should always be positive. It is good to repeat: "*Everything in my life has been changing for the better.*" Repeating these words for one to two minutes every day will lead to visible results.

There are periods during the day when positive affirmations work more effectively. Such times are at night before going to sleep and in the morning when you have just woken up, because the body at these times is most relaxed, breathing is quiet, and every cell and every nerve in your body is able to "hear" and absorb the content of your thoughts.

It is understood that your last thoughts before going to sleep work in your mind all night. If before falling asleep you say to yourself *"I am so tired,"* *"I am so unhappy,"* or *"I am so sick,"* these negative statements will dwell in your brain throughout the night, and in the morning when you wake up your thoughts may prove to have been keen and accurate predictions even though you have rested and should have more energy. Instead, it is better to repeat positive affirmations before going to sleep, such as *"In my sleep I become better, stronger and healthier,"* *"I am at peace, I am calm,"* or *"In the morning I will wake up in a good mood and in better health."* One or two of these affirmations should be your last thoughts before you fall asleep. In the morning as you awaken and your body is still relaxed and your eyes are still closed, say to yourself, one or two of these:

"Today I will have a good day"
"I'm full of energy"
"I am confident in myself"
"I'm calm"
"I love myself"
"I am free"
"I am able to cope with any problems"

Try to work out a new, more positive view of yourself even if you do not believe in it yet. Our brain usually works habitually, and if you have a limited, negative opinion of yourself, it is deep-rooted in your mind, so try to replace it by developing new positive thoughts. Repeat them for days and weeks or as long as is needed to completely replace the old negative attitudes.

Our life is usually full of stress, frustrations, heartaches, losses, and challenges and we must be careful because these negative influences may just pull us "down to the bottom." American writer Robert Frost said that it is important to strengthen positive self-esteem and maintain a healthy self-image:

> *"Timid thoughts create a timid man.*
> *Positive thoughts create a confident man.*
> *Weak thoughts create a weak-willed man.*
> *Strong thoughts create a strong man.*
> *Self-pity creates a man who will always feel*
> *sorry for himself.*
> *Sympathy creates a loving person, etc."*

Each person is responsible for creating and maintaining a relationship with him- or herself. The relationship depends on the attitude, positive or negative, you have toward *you*. Some people were not lucky or happy in childhood and adolescence—forget about it—you must live in the present moment. Looking back and remembering past troubles and distresses increases unhappiness in the present. You should be grateful and forgiving to yourself. Thinking too much about the future may bring more doubts and fears about our ability to overcome the current troubles in your life. The only thing you should take into account is how and what you think about now, in the present moment, and what you intend, on the mind level, to do in the future, not including emotions. It is very important to work on changing your attitude and be mindful of how everything has changed within and around you. Thus, everything is in our hands.

The Dalai Lama was asked what amazed him most. He said: "Man. At first, he sacrifices his health in order to make money. Then he spends the money to restore his health. At the same time he is so worried about his future, he never enjoys the present. As a result, he does not live either in the present or in the future. He lives as if he will never die, and dying regrets that he never lived."

It is important to perceive stress and problems as opportunities and challenges, not as obligations or obstacles. Yoga teaches that inner calmness strengthens the will, helps overcome difficulties, and saves energy.

156

Hippocrates said that reason and motivation are the best healers.

In yoga each person is understood to be special, unique and worthy of respect. Everyone is a star, and everyone you meet on your life path also is a star. When you talk with somebody, learn to look deeply into his or her soul. Greatness and uniqueness can be found within each individual. You should give people a chance because behind their failings and problems you can find their potential, their soul, their inner beauty and talents.

It is very important to develop positive thinking in everyday life, practicing spiritual yoga helps to develop and actualize the right attitudes in your life. Mechanically repeating affirmations only brings minimal results. Ideally, you do affirmations not to convince yourself of something but to bring your mind to a higher level of being. In essence, you are already at this level; you just need to progress and deepen your knowledge, and develop abilities for self-help and self-healing. When you repeat affirmations with a deep feeling of necessity, and with an open mind and heart, you understand that you can control your mind, and the affirmations bring you extraordinary power.

To do this next exercise, sit on a chair, keep your back upright; take several minutes to relax your breathing, body, emotions and mind. Suppose you've chosen the affirmation "*I am healthy, I am strong*." Visualize yourself young and healthy, and hold this vision. You can recall yourself when you were young and healthy, or you can look at a photo from your best period of life. Next, imagine that your body is filled with energy, imagine that you are getting stronger—your eyes shine, your muscles and body are strong and flexible, you have no pain, and your heart is filled with happiness and joy. When you repeat "*I am filled with energy,*" imagine yourself when you were strong and energetic, visualize light and energy filling your whole body, each muscle, and each nerve. Practicing visualization and concentration of mind several minutes every day will really help you feel better and be stronger physically and emotionally.

Every human being lives on several levels at the same time: physical, emotional, mental, and spiritual. Yogic wisdom teaches that the spiritual level is the most important. "The spirit" is called by different names—the soul, the essence of an individual (the Self), the light, the divine nature of God. Every person intuitively knows and feels that she is made up of more than just a body, character and personality. The higher spiritual level is in each of us, but we often do not realize it, though we feel intuitively that some higher reality exist beyond us. The goal of yoga is to develop and increase intuition, and to create balance with the higher level of our existence.

It is very important to find some time during the day (from 5-10 minutes) to practice yoga breathing exercises to calm the mind and emotions; and then to release tension by practicing deep relaxation and healing meditation. Although I have said this before, I repeat it here to emphasize the importance of yoga for spiritual well-being.

The power of forgiveness

Forgiveness is one of the most important aspects of human life. Swami Kriyananda [19, pp. 107 -109], talking about forgiveness, said that if you remember having ever hurt anybody, mentally send him blessings. If you've desecrated your own higher self-image, face that memory frankly, but calmly and dispassionately. If you've ever held negative thoughts toward anyone, send him blessings; raise your feeling to a level where you find yourself thinking of that person with kindness. If ever you've spoken critically of, or mocked anyone even mentally, offer him now your heartfelt kindness and good wishes for his eventual wisdom and inner freedom.

Colin Tipping [18] says that we human beings are very sensitive. Generally, people are vulnerable and easily hurt. When a person suffers an insult, he sometimes wants to inflict pain on others because of the common belief that blame is simply a way of life. Usually, when somebody is hurt, abused, deceived, or betrayed, he believes that someone has mistreated him, and this someone is directly responsible for his unhappiness in life. Some people have a tendency to blame others for their own failures and bad experiences. People begin to feel that they are victims of circumstance. Colin Tipping calls this "victim consciousness."

Some people, when they are experiencing fears, frustrations, and difficulties, often try to splash all these negative feelings onto relatives, close friends and acquaintances. Therefore, when you feel hurt or offended, it is so important to ask yourself what pain the offender is experiencing. Look into his soul with compassion and love. In his book, Tipping describes a special program that helps people develop to this level of relationship.

Sometimes we forget that our most intimate relationship is our relationship with ourselves. Sometimes we forget that everyone is a special person, very unique and deserving of respect. In his book "Radical Forgiveness," Mr. Tipping explains what True Forgiveness really means:

that there are no good, bad, right or wrong actions—it's simply our thoughts and beliefs that make them so. The power of forgiveness is effective to the extent to which it appeals to the highest human qualities such as tolerance, kindness, mercy, and humility. It is these qualities in us that inspire us to forgive and therefore have some healing potential.

It is most important to forgive ourselves for our "bad" actions toward people in the past and present. True forgiveness is entirely dependent on our ability to be compassionate, but our ego and personality are often looking for someone to blame. If someone has offended, humiliated, or betrayed us, it means that this person has deeply suffered in his soul in the past. And though it may be difficult for us to feel compassion for him and not take offense, we end up storing our grievance for years—and that may damage our physical or emotional health. Spiritual yoga teaches us that we should not only sympathize with others but we should mentally send offenders wishes of health and peace. This helps us remain internally protected from negative responses. It is also crucial to be patient with and kind to yourself, especially if you hurt or offended someone, offer yourself the same compassion of forgiveness.

Look ahead with hope, look back gratefully, above with belief, and look around with love.

Indian proverb

HEALING MEDITATION

Parable of the Lost Wristwatch

A man was frantically searching for something in a dark room. He was weeping and shouting. He was making a mess of the things kept in the room. He broke some and stumbled on others. Yet, what he was searching for, he could not find.

A friend came to the threshold and asked the reason for the man's misery. He replied: "O my friend, I have lost my wrist-watch. It is gone. The friend said: "How can it have disappeared by itself? But, what a fool you are to search for it in the dark! I have brought a light. Now, calm yourself. Think deeply and try to remember where it ought to be. You will soon discover it."

The man did so, and found the wrist-watch. The friend explained: "The watch was not lost, nor have you found it just now. It was there all the time. But because of the darkness that prevailed in the room, and because you were searching for it where it was not, you did not find it. You were ignorant of its whereabouts. Now that the ignorance is removed, you think you have got it. Yet it was never yours and it was never lost."

Similarly, within the deepest recesses of man's heart is the Self, full of bliss and peace. But, blinded by the darkness of ignorance, man is unable to see it and experience the bliss and the peace. Searching for happiness and peace, he wanders about among the objects of this world, makes a mess of himself and the things of the world, and causes misery to others and to himself, weeping and shouting. But the object of his quest is not found. At last the Teacher appears with the lamp of wisdom in his hand. He says to the man: "Remove the darkness of your ignorance with this lamp of wisdom; calm yourself. Then analyze all experience and meditate on the result. You will discover the Self. You had not lost it before; nor have you gained it now. It has always been there. Only you were ignorant of it. Now that in your pure heart and calm mind, the Self shines, self-

luminous, you feel that you have regained it. In fact you had never lost it. "

Meditation is the heart of yoga practice. It is a calm quiet state where there is no worry or confusion. Meditation calms the emotions and strengthens the nerves. When the mind is quiet, we open a channel to our Higher Self. People do not usually bring awareness to everyday life. They function simply by habit.

There are different techniques of meditation and all of them help you be more aware of yourself and aware of life around you. Healing Meditation is accessible for both people who are healthy and those who have some health problems [6,8, 10,14, 25, 26, 27].

Suffering on the physical, emotional, or mental level is often increased by negative thinking about oneself, like: "*I'm never going to get better. My life is over. Nobody's going to want me now. I am so unhappy.*" In other words, negative thoughts create negative emotions, and negative attitudes prevent a person from self-healing.

Meditation is an ancient yoga technique for self-healing and self-improvement. Studies by psychologists have determined that meditation can increase your mood, decrease anxiety, and increases your attention. Meditation also strengthens your sense of well-being, confidence, clarity, gratitude and compassion. On a physical level, meditation strengthens the immune system. It helps you also to be aware of the present moment, connect your sense of self to your moment-to-moment experience, which, ultimately, helps you enjoy your life.

It is important to meditate in a sitting position, keeping your back, neck and head aligned. If you bend slightly forward, you may fall asleep. To help keep the back supported and upright, place a pillow or folded blanket at the lower back. If you feel that it is difficult for you to meditate while sitting in a chair, you can meditate in lying position.

Ideally, meditation requires a strong body and spine. This is one of the reasons that practicing yoga postures, breathing exercises and deep relaxation are so important—because they strengthen the whole body—and this helps avoid stiffness and tension during meditation. Therefore, it's best to wait until you feel physically comfortable and able meditating, in either a sitting or lying position, for at least 10-15 minutes.

It is up to you to decide when you are ready to begin doing the healing meditations. Do you have a strong desire or aspiration to meditate? Or do you feel you that you don't really need it? If you feel that you do not need to practice meditation that is okay—just focus on the breathing and relaxation exercises instead. When you feel that you are ready, find 10-15 minutes during the day (morning is best) for meditation. It is important to be in a room alone, with the phone turned off and, if possible, nothing else to disturb or distract you.

Sit in a chair or lie on your back. Close your eyes and focus your mind on observing your body. Next, begin slowly relaxing each muscle in your body, going through the body from the feet to the head consciously releasing all tension. Relax your emotions and your mind, and keep breathing through the diaphragm. Feel your body completely relaxed, and mentally look up, relaxing your eyes and eyelids. Now bring your attention to your breath itself, calmly feeling its flow in and out through your nostrils. Feel the cool air in your nostrils as you inhale, and warm air as you exhale. This simple exercise helps calm your mind and emotions and brings you into a deeper sense of relaxation. Continue your diaphragmatic breathing, keeping it quiet and rhythmical. In several minutes, as you exhale, choose one or two affirmations and repeat each 4-5 times: *"I am at peace,"* *"I am relaxed,"* *"I am Light,"* or *"I am Love."* Hold a very short pause after each repetition, feeling and enjoying the peace, calmness and love.

Slowly, with patience and practice, your mind will become more relaxed, calmer, and more peaceful.

166

Advanced level yoga teachings describe meditation as reaching a higher state of consciousness. But that takes long and regular practice. In the beginning thoughts will usually arise in the mind, but you should calmly bring them back to the point of focus—to feelings of calmness, peace, and light.

There are numerous scenarios for meditation. Below I present three simple nature scenarios; you should choose the one that you are most drawn to. Or you can try all of them in turn.

The first scenario: When you are deeply relaxed and your mind is calm, imagine yourself sitting on the beach near the ocean. Imagine that no one is around, you are sitting on the warm, soft sand,. Visualize the endless ocean in front of you, and "see" the calm surface of ocean, "hear" the soft waves that are lap at the shore. Now mentally look up, relaxing your eyes and eyelids, and consciously observe the endless blue sky. Imagine light all around you and be present in the deep silence, the peace and joy within and around you. Stay here as long as is comfortable. When you feel ready, take a deep breath, open your eyes, and slowly come out of the meditation. Take some time to notice how you felt before meditation and compare it to how you feel now. Even doing short meditations you will start to feel a positive difference—you will notice an increase in energy and balance, and feel calmer, both emotionally and mentally.

The second scenario: You are sitting or lying near a big shade tree. Imagine in front of you a big green meadow filled with bright flowers. Enjoy the scent of flowers. The sun's rays break through the crowns and leaves of the tree, and they glow and warm you. Nobody is around. You enjoy the peace and beauty surrounding you and feel your whole body filled with energy and light. You feel deep peace in your heart. Stay here as long as is comfortable. When you finish take several deep breaths and come out of the meditation.

The third scenario: Close your eyes and imagine yourself sitting on top of a very high mountain. Imagine the clear blue sky above you. Notice how the light surrounds you on all sides. You can see the endless ridges of the many hills below. You breathe fresh mountain air, and enjoy the stunning view. You begin to notice that your body, mind and emotions are completely relaxed and calm. And now feel the deep peace, love and joy that fill your heart. Stay here as long as you like. When you are ready, take a deep breath and open your eyes.

When you meditate on one of the scenarios described above, imagine yourself outside of the everyday world. Close the door of your mind to all outside things, and immerse yourself in the vast, silent world within.

Meditation is often viewed as just a way to relax—and that's all. But in truth it is a very specific practice of deep concentration and attention on the Higher Self, Spirit, or on the Essence of the Universe that helps you to learn to be detached from your health and emotional problems. It nourishes the root of your personality, your nervous system, and your mind by use of subtle energy and light, like a nourishing food, making you healthier, stronger and happier.

Some people like to meditate alone, but for others it is easier to meditate in a group. So you might be better off looking for a meditation group in your area. Anyone can practice meditation spending even a few minutes a day at it to restore your calmness and inner peace.

I recall when I began to meditate in the early 1970s, how difficult it was for me to calm my mind. My spiritual teacher said one day that I was too stressed and had a lot of anxiety, and these made it difficult for me to improve my ability to follow the spiritual path of yoga. He recommended that I meditate every day and advised me to organize and discipline myself. I came to meditation practice seriously, focusing on deep relaxation and quiet breathing, and slowly that helped me to relax my mind and emotions. I prayed to something existing beyond me for help and guidance to deepen my meditation. With everyday practice I learned to concentrate and focus my attention on peace, light and joy. In the beginning it was not easy; the hardest moments, as I remember, were the thoughts that sprang up one after another. Gradually the flow of thoughts slowed and I began to enjoy inner calmness, mental stillness and inner silence. I tried to imagine Light and Peace within and around me, and finished meditation by praying for protection for my family and myself and for help in being healthier and stronger.

Under the guidance of my teacher, I followed the path of Kriya Yoga and aspired to self-realization. The path of self-realization was revealed in America by Paramahansa Yogananda, who was a Master of spiritual yoga, philosopher and psychologist, and who came to America from India in 1929. Swami Kriyananda was the foremost, direct disciple of Paramhansa Yogananda in the 1940s and the early 1950s. Later he became the spiritual director and founder of the Ananda Spiritual Center located in California. Swami Kriyananda developed an important aspect of Paramahansa Yogananda's work—the creation of spiritual communities where people could live according to the principles of spiritual yoga. I have learned from the writings of Paramahansa Yogananda and Swami

Kriyananda that meditation requires great spiritual effort and a strong will. This is especially true in the beginning when you are learning to practice yoga postures, breathing exercises and relaxation, and affirmations. I paid a lot of attention to reading the spiritual literature and learned that this path requires a deep faith and patience, systematic discipline, and, most importantly, regular meditation. I have been on this path for more than 40 years and feel how, with practice, I have become more peaceful emotionally, stronger mentally, and more spiritually uplifted.

Paramahansa Yogananda told us that harmony comes from within as natural fulfillment. A person who cannot understand himself cannot understand others. A person should first feel at home with himself and then he will be able to find harmony in interaction with everyone who comes into contact with him. S. Kriyananda in his book "God is for Everyone" wrote that his teacher P.Yogananda taught his students to understand and realize eight aspects of God as Essence of the Universe: Love, Wisdom, Peace, deep Calmness, Power, Joy, Light, and Sound [3, pp.209 – 210], he also added that wisdom is the direct perception of the Truth.

Swami Kriyananda told us that realization of these aspects brings happiness [3, p.50] and that happiness springs from within the self. It does not depend on outer conditions. Nothing outside ourselves, therefore, can define our happiness except as we allow it to do so. Once the truth is realized, happiness becomes our permanent possession. Unfortunately, people seek fulfillment mostly in outside life conditions, not inside, in themselves.

Truth is a complex word. Truth lies in a constant feeling of happiness. It means that permanent happiness refers not to temporary sharp sensations that accompany material success and fun, but in the joy found only in the union of the individual soul with God, or Spirit. Yogananda showed that there are three ways to attain truth: through perception, reasoning, and also through intuition. He added that only through the development of intuition can a man learn what the truth is.

Intuition is a direct or immediate perception; it is pure omniscient awareness of the soul. Yogananda believed that the only way to know and live in truth is to develop the power of intuition. The best way to develop intuition is through meditation.

Joy is explained, by its nature, as blissful consciousness of the Spirit in the human soul. It springs down the mind and is born in it when its source is internal. In contrast to material pleasures, true Joy is not an abstract quality of mind; it is conscious, and expresses itself in the quality of the Spirit. Joy means inspirational spiritual uplift, the expression of Supreme Bliss.

Yogananda told us that Love is a natural feeling of the soul, but in relation to Joy it is secondary. Love cannot exist without Joy. Joy goes together with Love. When we speak about the suffering of unreciprocated love, it means we have an unfulfilled desire. True love is always filled with joy. Love is given without expecting anything in return. Yogananda emphasized that love cannot be obtained upon request; it only comes as a gift from the heart.

The longer you meditate, the more likely you will begin to feel Love and Joy in your heart. When you meditate regularly you will wish to meditate longer.

Healing meditation helps you receive many advantages such as increased self-control over fear, anxiety, negative thoughts, and mood swings, and the ability to be calm, relaxed, and happy at all times.

Just before meditation, pray to God, or Infinite Spirit, or to your Higher Self, or, if you like, to whomever or whatever exists beyond you, and ask for good health, strength, and wisdom. Ask for guidance in deep meditation. The meaning and power of prayer will come to you with practice.

At the end of meditation pray again. You can say *"Thank you for healing presence, for guiding in every moment of my life,"* or *"Lead me from darkness to light."*

The spiritual experience is an awareness of and relationship with something that goes beyond your personal self as well as the human order of things. The word *spiritual* brings up the wonderful nature of the energy that comes from an invisible, intelligent source. The healing energy from this source is available to all.

Spirituality brings you to a sense of humility, liberation, trust, order, and the ability to stay grounded despite the regular instability and changes in the world. Through yoga, and the spiritual component of yoga, you can come into direct contact with joy, happiness, love and compassion.

Religious people believe in God and pray to Him. Spiritual people, who usually do not belong to a particular religion, have a faith in cosmic consciousness, or the infinite Spirit, revealed as Higher Self, as the wisdom of Higher Power, Universal Subtle Energy, or Essence of Universe, and also as Love, Light and Joy.

"There is no need for temples; no need for complicated philosophy. Our own brain, our own heart is our temple."

Dalai Lama

Paramahansa Yogananda said in his work *Divine Will Healing: The Law of Divine Healing:* "Remember that doubt, mental fatigue, worry, indifference, boredom, fear, restlessness, timidity, mental and physical laziness, over-indulgence, unmethodical life, lack of interest, and lack of creative ability are counteracting static agents which make it impossible for the cosmic energy to tune in with man.

"...Creative spiritual ambition, calmness, and courage, unconquered attitude, tolerance, patience, and peace are avenues through which cosmic energy can help you.

This is a great secret law that some know, but few put into actual practice. If you continuously persist in thinking that your body is full of vitality, especially at a time when it is weak, then you will find that you have started to open up a new secret, invisible source of vitalizing yourself other than from the external material sources of food, and so forth."

A prayer from *Bhagavad Gita [3]:*

"Supreme God, your light is brighter than the sun, your purity whiter than mountain snow; you are present wherever I go. Show me how I can meditate upon you, learning from you the wisdom that I need. I am never tired of hearing you, because your words bring life. Give me strength for today, and hope for tomorrow."

Many people feel the need to pray only when they are suffering from fear, are in strong pain or are in other emergency situations. They ask Higher Power to help them in this difficult moment and they hope to receive relief.

Sincere prayer, however, offers faith and love and comes from a deep desire for Spirit's guidance, healing and protection. In deep prayer to a Higher Power you receive great inspiration and guidance to Love, Light and healing. Faith is a very powerful resource.

Meditation and Prayer are not a religion, philosophy, or lifestyle. It's the most widely practiced and most effective method of self-development and self-healing.

"Your vision will become clear only when you look into your heart." St. Therese of Lisieux

"... Who looks outside, dreams. Who looks inside, awakens." Carl Jung

People who don't believe in God, but still feel a curiosity or pull toward prayer can use the Loving-Kindness Prayer from Buddhism. According to Hogen Bays, a priest in the Zen Community of Oregon:

"The function of prayer is to connect us with that which is greater than our small self."

May I be free from fear.
May I be free from suffering.
May I be happy.
May I be filled with loving-kindness.

The basic idea behind most forms of meditation is to focus the mind on turning inward, to pay attention to your inner self so that your mind is open and clear. Prayer is essentially the exact opposite of meditation. During prayer you focus your thoughts on the prayer itself and the answers you hope to find by praying. In essence, we meditate so that Spirit can speak to us; we pray so that we can speak to Spirit.

Two wolves

Once upon a time an old man told his grandson a vital truth: -"In every man there is a struggle going on inside, much like a terrible fight between two wolves. One wolf is evil; he is anger, envy, jealousy, sorrow, regret, greed, ambition, guilt, inferiority, lies, and self-doubt. The other wolf is good; he is joy, peace, love, hope, truth, hope, serenity, humility, kindness, empathy, generosity, truth, compassion, and faith. This same fight is going on inside you, and inside every other person, too."

The grandson, touched to the heart by the words of his grandfather, thought about it for a minute, and then asked his grandfather, "Which wolf will win in the end?" The old man smiled and replied simply, "The one you feed."

To become conscious of the greatness, strength and power of your real being is certainly worth months or years of the often-challenging study and practice of yoga postures, breathing, relaxation, and meditation.

If you have some physical limitations or emotional problems try to do at least a little something, choosing what would be easiest for you at this time—try some postures, or you can start out by practicing only the relaxation and breathing exercises, or even just the positive self-suggestions for strengthening your mind. When you feel ready, begin to practice healing meditation and healing prayer. With practice you will intuitively feel your body's possibilities and abilities for self-improvement and self-healing.

After working with this book you may be able to find yoga classes or meditation groups in your area. There are also classes and interesting information and support on line.

"I will with my own will, which flows from the Divine Will, to be healthy, to be well, to be prosperous and spiritual, to be well, and to be well."

Affirmation of Paramhansa Yogananda

SUGGESTED READING

1. AFFIRMATIONS for Self-Healing, by J. Donald Walters (Swami Kriyananda); Crystal Clarity Publishers, Nevada City, CA (2005).

2. Autobiography of a Yogi by Paramhansa Yogananda; Crystal Clarity Publishers, Nevada City, CA (1996).

3. AYURVEDA; The Science of Self-Healing, a practical guide by Dr. Vasant Lad; Lotus Light, Wilmot, WI (1990).

4. GOD IS FOR EVERYONE, inspired by Paramhansa Yogananda; as taught to and understood by his disciple, J. Donald Walters (Swami Kriyananda); Crystal Clarity Publishers, Nevada City, CA (2003).
This is the core of Yogananda's teachings. The book presents a concept of God and spiritual meaning that will broadly appeal to everyone, agnostics and believers alike.

5. HEALING YOGA FOR PEOPLE LIVING WITH CANCER by Lisa Holtby; Taylor Trade Publishing, NY (2004).

6. HOW TO ACHIEVE GLOWING HEALTH AND VITALITY by Paramahansa Yogananda; Crystal Clarity Publishers, Nevada City, CA (2010).

7. HOW TO HAVE COURAGE, CALMNESS AND CONFIDENCE. The Wisdom of Paramhansa Yogananda, Volume 5; Crystal Clarity Publishers, Nevada City, CA (2010).

If you are facing challenges in your life right now, know that you have within you all that you need to rise to meet them, and to deal with them in the best way possible.

8. HOW TO BE HAPPY ALL THE TIME. The Wisdom of Paramhansa Yogananda, Volume 1;

Crystal Clarity Publishers, Nevada City, CA (2006)

The human drive for happiness is one of our most far-reaching and fundamental needs. Yet, it seems that very few of us have truly unlocked the secrets of lasting joy and inner peace.

9. HOW TO BE A SUCCESS; the Wisdom of Paramhansa Yogananda Volume 4. Crystal Clarity Publishers, Nevada City, CA. (2008)

There is a power that can reveal hidden veins of riches and uncover treasures of which we never dreamed.

10. HOW TO MEDITATE, by Jyotish Novak, A Step-by-Step Guide to the Art & Science of Meditation; Crystal Clarity Publishers, Nevada City, CA, (2008).
This bestselling revised and expanded book presents a thorough yet concise step-by-step guide to the art and science of meditation.

11. FREEDOM FROM STRESS, How to Take Control of Your Life; by David Gamow with Karen Gamow, Published by Glenbridge Publishing Ltd., Centennial, Colorado 2006

12. LIVING WISELY, LIVING WELL, Timeless Wisdom to Enrich Every Day, by Swami Kriyananda; Crystal Clarity Publishers, Nevada City, CA (1911).

13. MAYO CLINIC ON ARTHRITIS, by Gene Hunder, M.D. Mayo Clinic, Rochester, MN (2002).

14. MEDITATION FOR STARTERS, by J. Donald Walters (Swami Kriyananda); Cristal Clarity Publishers, Nevada City, CA (1996).

15. NATURAL HEALTH, NATURAL MEDICINE, by Andrew Weil, M.D., A comprehensive manual for wellness and self-care, Houghton Mifflin Company, Boston (1990).

16. YOGA THERAPY FOR OVERCOMING INSOMNIA, by Peter Van Houten, M.D. & Gyandev Rich McCord, Ph.D., Crystal Clarity Publishers, Nevada City, CA (2004).

17. PEACE, LOVE AND HEALING, by Bernie Siegel; HarperCollins, New York, NY (1990).

18. RADICAL FORGIVENESS, by Colin Tipping. Sounds True, Boulder, CO (2009).

19. RELIGION IN THE NEW AGE AND OTHER ESSAYS FOR THE SPIRITUAL SEEKER, Swami Kriyananda, Cristal Clarity Publishers, Nevada City, CA (2009).

20. STRETCH AND RELAX, by Maxim Tobias & Mary Stewart; the Body Press, Tucson, AZ (1985).

21. STRETCH AND SURRENDER: A GUIDE TO YOGA, HEALTH AND RELAXATION FOR PEOPLE IN RECOVERY, Annalisa Cunningham. Rudra Press, Portland, Oregon (1992).

22. STOP PAIN: INFLAMMATION RELIEF FOR AN ACTIVE LIFE by Vijay Vad M.D., 2011

23. YOGA THERAPY FOR HEADACHE RELIEF, by Peter van Houten, MD, and Nayaswami Gyandev McCord (Gyandev Rich McCord, Ph.D.); Crystal Clarity Publishers, Nevada City, CA (2004).

Topics covered include: the different types of headaches and how to tell them apart; how yoga can help relieve them; two safe, effective routines—one short, the other longer—detailing which yoga postures to use for best results; additional alternative techniques that may be helpful.

RESOURSES

24. THE AYURVEDIC REHABILITATION CENTER

Loretta Levitz – Director; David Liberty – Assistant Director; specializing in WHOLE HEALTH TRAINING

INDIVIDUALIZED PROGRAMS – Ayurvedic Constitutional Analysis; Therapeutic Touch; Ayurvedic Nutrition; Personalized Yoga Programs; Polarity, HATHA YOGA CLASSES, 617-782-1727; 105 Bennett St. Brighton, MA 01235

25. MEDITATION THERAPY FOR STRESS AND CHANGE, DVD, by Jyotish Novak (author of "How to Meditate"; www.crystalclarity.com;

Meditation Therapy is a bold new approach to finding lasting solutions to our deepest problems and concerns. Combining the power of deep meditation practice with the insights of psychology will help you enrich your life in lasting ways.

26. RELAX: MEDITATIONS FOR FLUTE AND CELLO, Sharon Brooks & David Eby. This CD is specifically designed to slow respiration and heart rate, bringing listeners to their calm center; www.crystalclarity.com

27. RELAX: MEDITATION WITH PIANO MUSIC, David Miller.

"Let peace gently enfold you as you listen to these lilting melodies. This soothing instrumental music is the perfect antidote to stress of all types. Calming and inspiring, it will lift you above day-to-day worries and cares. Play it after work, before falling asleep or anytime you want to banish tensions and troubles." www.crystalclarity.com

28. Visit the website www.ananda.org where you can find classes, articles and support information; they also classes in Healing Prayer, Tools for Spiritual Living, and retreats.

29. YOGA FOR EMOTIONAL HEALTH by Lisa Powers, Bringing Balance, Inner Peace, & Happiness into Your Life DVD, 85 minutes

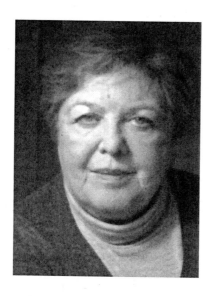

About the Author

Anna Shapiro, as psychologist and psychotherapist for 45 years, as a Yoga teacher of 35 years, as well as a yoga therapist for last 20 years. Born in Russia, Moscow, in 1941, where persecution and the fear of persecution were realities of her daily life there.

Anna practiced Yoga since 1968. At that time in Soviet Russia Yoga was referred to as "health improvement classes" because Yoga was considered a form of foreign propaganda due to its message of true spiritual freedom, which went against the country's political ideology.

While still in Russia, in 1970 Anna met a Yoga teacher who guided her in theory and practice of meditation and yoga philosophy, which in turn helped her to deepen her understanding of a spiritual path. He helped her to understand the subtle inner world of intuition and how to meditate on the different aspects of God.

In 1979 Anna's family applied for permission to leave Russia, as Soviet Russia at the time was a closed society and no one could leave its borders without obtaining such permission first. Unfortunately, the family was refused to leave Russia. As the government punished everyone who wanted to leave Russia in some way, Anna and her husband were forced from their jobs and were not allowed to be hired elsewhere. They lived every day under the surveillance of the KGB. Thus began the family's long and painful wait for a possible permission to leave Russia, which lasted for ten years. During this period, the family's life was a mixture of uncertainty and fear of arrest, financial struggle, overshadowed, however, with the will and determination to overcome all difficulties.

In 1975 Anna Shapiro began to teach yoga at home, she had to hold her classes secretly because officially it was prohibited and could be punished by imprisonment. Some of her original students are still in contact with her and continue to practice Yoga and its principles.

Finally, at the end of 1988, the family at last received a permission to leave Russia and in the late Spring of that year, Anna, her husband, daughter and father have arrived to Boston area.

While in US, Anna became certified in Yoga and as an Ayurveda practitioner. For many years she has also worked as a psychotherapist for the Jewish Family and Children's Services in Boston from 1994 until her retirement in 2004. In the last few years she has been teaching Yoga classes for people over 50 and continues to provide individual and group yogatherepy.

In yoga practice Anna combines her extensive experience as a psychologist and as a yoga teacher, and that gives her a unique profile in helping her students on a deeper level. She has been asked to give public lectures on numerous occasions on such topics as "Yoga and Stress Management," "Yoga and Pain Control," and "Yoga and Self-Healing."

Her first book, memoirs entitled "Threads of Fate" was published in Boston in 2012.